Ngā Kūaha

Ngā Kūaha: Voices and Visions in Māori Healing and Psychiatry explores what it means to hear voices and see visions from the perspectives of Māori healer Wiremu NiaNia and psychiatrist Allister Bush. Wiremu explains Ngā Kūaha as referring to doorways and offers entranceways into Māori knowledge about wairua (spirituality) handed down by his forebears and other Māori sources.

The authors provide historical examples of Western mystical experiences and contrasting Western psychiatric and psychological explanations of voices and visions as hallucinations. Further chapters focus on narratives and perspectives from people who have experienced voices and visions, and have had interactions with mental health services, told from multiple viewpoints; individual, whānau (family), Māori healing and psychiatry. The benefits of joint Māori healing and psychiatry approaches on wellbeing are examined. Drawing on their 18-year partnership, Wiremu and Allister highlight the harmful colonial impact of psychiatry in suppressing Māori views of voices and visions. They describe ways of working together in clinical practice to address this history of injustice and how to identify whether distressing perceptual experiences may represent Māori cultural experiences, psychiatric or psychological symptoms or all of these.

This book advocates for practices that enable genuine partnerships between Māori healers, other wairua practitioners and mental health clinicians in order to improve the mental health and spiritual care of Māori and perhaps other peoples.

Wiremu NiaNia, Tohunga, Turuki Health Care, Tāmaki-makau-rau Auckland, Aotearoa New Zealand.

Allister Bush, Child and Adolescent Psychiatrist, Te Whare Mārie, Māori Mental Health Service and Pasifika CAMHS (Child and Adolescent Mental Health Service), Te Whatu Ora, Porirua, Aotearoa New Zealand.

David Epston, Co-originator of Narrative Therapy, Tāmaki-makau-rau Auckland, Aotearoa New Zealand.

Writing Lives

Ethnographic and Autoethnographic Narratives

Series Editors: Arthur P. Bochner, Carolyn Ellis, and Tony E. Adams

University of South Florida and Bradley University

Writing Lives: Ethnographic and Autoethnographic Narratives publishes narrative representations of qualitative research projects. The series editors seek manuscripts that blur the boundaries between humanities and social sciences. We encourage novel and evocative forms of expressing concrete lived experience, including autoethnographic, literary, poetic, artistic, visual, performative, critical, multi-voiced, conversational, and co-constructed representations. We are interested in ethnographic narratives that depict local stories; employ literary modes of scene setting, dialogue, character development, and unfolding action; and include the author's critical reflections on the research and writing process, such as research ethics, alternative modes of inquiry and representation, reflexivity, and evocative storytelling. Proposals and manuscripts should be directed to abochner@usf.edu, cellis@usf.edu or tadams@bradley.edu

Writing Philosophical Autoethnography
Alec Grant

Unraveling
An Autoethnography of Suicide and Renewal
M.F. Alvarez

No One Can Arrest Our Dreams
Black Men Storying a Path Towards Educational Justice and Freedom
Clarice O. Thomas

White Folks
Race and Identity in Rural America, 2nd Edition
Timothy J. Lensmire

Ngā Kūaha
Voices and Visions in Māori Healing and Psychiatry
Wiremu NiaNia, Allister Bush, David Epston

For more information about this series, please visit:
www.routledge.com/Writing-Lives-Ethnographic-Narratives/book-series/WLEN

Ngā Kūaha

Voices and Visions in Māori Healing and Psychiatry

Wiremu NiaNia, Allister Bush, David Epston

Routledge
Taylor & Francis Group
NEW YORK AND LONDON

Designed cover image: 'Te Putanga o te Ao' (The Emergence of the World) by Tangi.

First published 2025
by Routledge
605 Third Avenue, New York, NY 10158

and by Routledge
4 Park Square, Milton Park, Abingdon, Oxon, OX14 4RN

Routledge is an imprint of the Taylor & Francis Group, an informa business

ISBN: 978-1-032-03380-8 (hbk)
ISBN: 978-1-032-03384-6 (pbk)
ISBN: 978-1-003-18704-2 (ebk)

DOI: 10.4324/9781003187042

Typeset in Optima
by SPi Technologies India Pvt Ltd (Straive)

For Product Safety Concerns and Information please contact our EU representative: GPSR@taylorandfrancis.com
Taylor & Francis Verlag GmbH, Kaufingerstraße 24, 80331 München, Germany.

This book is dedicated to all those who courageously seek understanding of whatever they are going through, and all those who have generously given their stories that we might learn

Contents

Wiremu NiaNia and Allister Bush were jointly awarded the 2021 Mark Sheldon Prize from the Royal Australian and New Zealand College of Psychiatrists. This prize recognises noteworthy contributions to Indigenous mental health in either Australia or New Zealand.

Acknowledgements

Ahakoa te hūkerikeri a ngaru	Despite the turbulence of the waves
Ka ekea e te waka	They can be ridden by the waka
Mai i ngā ia tere a Tangaroa	From the currents of Tangaroa
Ki Te-Moana-tāpokopoko-a-Tāwhaki ki Aotearoa	To the southern oceans and shores of Aotearoa
Ka ūnga ki te ara o Hinekirikiri ka tae ki uta	Anchoring in the shallows of Hinekirikiri and then to the land
Nau mai e te ope tūārangi	Welcome to all those from afar
Kia tau kia taui	

Without our whānau, there would be no book. We mihi to our Pou (our whānau) who have remained constant during many changing faces of the water which this waka encountered during the journey of this book. To Lesley NiaNia, Ruth Diggins and Ann Epston, and to all our whānau – we mihi to you for your aroha, kaha, karakia, guidance and tautoko.

We gratefully acknowledge all those who have contributed to the writing of this book. We especially recognise the courage and generosity of those who agreed to share their stories so that others might benefit. We acknowledge all those from te iwi Māori. We acknowledge our contributors from Te Moana-nui-a-Kiwa, from Samoa, from Cook Islands and from Tokelau.

We acknowledge Tohunga Nick Tupara and Tohunga Rikki Solomon for their comments on Chapter 2. We are grateful to Taimalieutu Kiwi Tamasese for her guidance on many matters. Thank you to our psychiatrist advisors Pete Ellis, Joanna MacDonald and Alec MacDonald for their feedback on all the chapters.

We are very appreciative of the contribution of our editor Linley Boniface whose skill and gracious advice improved the text in many ways. We thank Art Bochner, our series editor, and Hannah Shakespeare and Adam Woods, our editors at Routledge. We acknowledge Lynda Godsiff for transcription mahi and Nigel Brooke for proofreading of te reo.

We acknowledge Stuff Limited for permission to publish material from their podcast 'Angels and Demons' in Chapter 5; Penguin for consent to use several quotes in Chapter 2 and Hearing Voices Network Aotearoa for permission to use the quote from Karlo Mila in Chapter 5.

We mihi to Helena Keyes, Cathy Diggins, Tim McCreanor, Tehseen Noorani, Rachel Liebert, Liz O'Connor, Liam O'Connor, David Chaplow, Tarquin Bush, Isaac Bush, Nicolas Davey, Emily Davey, Rachel Hayward, Richard Holt, Tom Flewett, Zoe Hawkins and Lynley McLay, for their comments on particular chapters. We acknowledge Maire Ransfield, and Rongo Larkin for their comments and Ngā Kaumātua o Te Whare Mārie for their tautoko. Ngā mihi ki a koutou katoa.

Cover image explanation

From the artist: 'This painting depicts the creation of the universe, with Papatūānuku (Earth Mother) in red and Ranginui (Sky Father) in blue. The figures in yellow represent their children, with Tāne's limbs, Tangaroa as a whale and Rūaumoko in between. The shape of the painting resembles a doorway, opening into the broad unknown, trusting your mana and your tīpuna to protect you; entering the vast realm of sacredness, creativity, information and love with utmost respect and gratitude'.

Mihi

Ko te mihi tuatahi ki Te Kaituku Oranga ki a tātou mō ngā manaakitanga ko uhia mai ki runga i a tātou. Tuarua ka mihi ki a rātou kua hipa ki te wāhi ngaro. Kei te mihi, kei te mihi, kei te mihi. Kei te mihi ki a rātou nā rātou i toro-te-nukuroa; ki runga Te Moana-nui-a-Kiwa me te mata o te whenua hoki.

Me te mihi hoki ki a koutou, nā koutou i koha mai i ngā wāhanga o to māua tuhingaroa kāre i tua atu! Me kī nā rātou nā koutou otirā nā tātou katoa.

Anei rā te mihi ki a koutou kua aro mai ki wā māua tuhinga kōrero e pā ana ki tā māua mahi ki te taha o ētahi o ngā whānau e whai huarahi ana.

Toitū te whakaaronui!

Our first mihi (greeting) is to the Creator who gives life to us, who adorns us with a cloak of blessing and protection. Secondly, we acknowledge all those that came before us and have now passed beyond the veil; who crossed vast distances over oceans and land so we might be where we are today. Next, we greet and thank all those from many walks of life who gifted their stories for this book. Their generosity cannot be measured. Finally, we mihi to you, the reader, for your interest in this work with people and families who seek understanding and wellness.

Let us strive for unity in our purpose!

1 Introduction

Wiremu NiaNia, Allister Bush, and David Epston

Wiremu

Ngā Kūaha

Allister, David and I have written this book to bring Māori cultural and spiritual perspectives to the challenge of understanding voices, visions and other perceptual experiences. We hope this will contribute to more appropriate mental health understanding and care for Māori individuals and whānau (families), as well as anyone interested in wairua (the spiritual realm). Western psychiatry has often conceptualised voices and visions as hallucinations, implying that they are by definition a hallmark of mental illness. Māori explanations in Aotearoa (New Zealand) have usually been silenced, just as Indigenous perspectives have in many other parts of the world, and this has been detrimental to the wellbeing of our peoples.

The Māori title of this book is Ngā Kūaha. Kūaha refers to a doorway or an entranceway. It suggests the possibility of looking through: seeing, hearing and experiencing a different space or even a different world. In te ao Māori (the Māori world), when someone sees something in wairua, sometimes people refer to that as the opening of a spiritual doorway or portal. Perhaps that opening has been invited. However, it can also happen uninvited. In this respect, Ngā Kūaha can refer to the many ways that people experience wairua.

A further meaning is that of a doorway into different realms of understanding or knowledge. Kūaha is also another word for kūwaha. Waha refers to the mouth. When I open my mouth to kōrero (talk) with you, I'm opening up a doorway to share knowledge that has been handed down from generation to generation. It may be tapu (sacred or forbidden) knowledge. I would hope it would be respected and not trampled on. Ngā Kūaha suggests an entranceway into a knowledge space that you may not otherwise have an opportunity to step into. By sharing this mātauranga or knowledge with you, I am treating you like a rangatira (respected elder).

DOI: 10.4324/9781003187042-1

When you arrive at someone's door, you don't just bowl on in. You knock and wait for the owner to answer the door. There is an expression, 'Ka kuhu tonu ia', which refers to the ability to do things your way, in your time. It's an expression of self-determination. In this book, we are sharing viewpoints from both Allister and my worldviews, though we each have respect for the other's perspective.

In our first book, *Collaborative and Indigenous Mental Health Therapy: Tātaihono – Stories of Māori Healing and Psychiatry*, we shared stories of Māori healing with young people who were suffering from spiritual distress which closely resembled psychiatric or psychological problems (NiaNia et al., 2017b). In our work together at Te Whare Mārie, a Māori mental health service, and Health Pasifika, a Pasifika mental health service, in Porirua, New Zealand, Allister as a Pākehā (New Zealand European) child and adolescent psychiatrist and I as a Māori cultural therapist showed how it was possible for psychiatry and Māori healing to work closely together in genuine partnership, and for people to benefit from both approaches. In *Tātaihono* we were seeking to create awareness of wairua (spirituality) so that everyone could have more tools for their toolkit and knowledge for their kete (basket), whether that be individuals, whānau (family) or mental health professionals (NiaNia et al., 2017b).

Allister and I worked together at Te Whare Mārie from 2005 to 2010. Since that time Allister continues his mahi (work) there, and I have worked as a Māori healer in other Māori services in Gisborne, on the east coast of New Zealand's North Island, and in Auckland, the country's biggest city. However, despite this geographical distance, we have continued to work closely together, developing our partnership and seeing young people and their whānau together when circumstances allow. It was in 2010 when I first suggested to Allister that we start writing about this work.

In this book, we share additional stories about people in distress who turned up to mental health services with experiences of seeing, hearing and feeling things that were not apparent to others. In some stories I describe my own experiences that were not perceived by others present to show how these experiences appeared to me. In each case, the people we met with benefited from a wairua healing approach alongside psychiatry. We will also examine the meanings of voices and visions from Māori perspectives alongside Western viewpoints, including psychology and psychiatry.

Many of my people in the past who were experiencing Māori cultural phenomena had their experiences interpreted by mental health professionals as psychiatric symptoms, resulting in inappropriate diagnosis and treatment. As a result, Māori who have experiences such as voices and visions may become very anxious that they have a mental health problem such as psychosis.

Throughout this book, we advocate for awareness of wairua and the impact it might have on a person's wellbeing. We ask mental health professionals to consider this when they are working with Māori whānau. In addition, we are suggesting that collaboration between Māori healing and psychiatry can provide whānau with more appropriate assessment and healing or treatment options than either approach can alone.

In this chapter Allister and I briefly describe our different backgrounds and the formative experiences that shaped our views on the meanings we give to voices and visions. I also introduce some of the ways I think about these often puzzling experiences from my perspective as a Māori healer.

Whāngai

I was born in 1949 in a woolshed in a rural area near Gisborne. I was the eighth of my mother's 16 children. As a result, several of us were adopted out as whāngai (extended family adoptees). I was given to my mother's niece, Nancy NiaNia, to raise. Nancy was 19 at the time but she died a year later, so I grew up with her mother, Te Awhimate. I called Te Awhimate Mum or Nan, but I usually refer to her as my kuia (female elder). Her father, William Trainor, was Welsh and became the local policeman in Rūātoki, a Māori settlement in the middle of the Ngāi Tūhoe tribal area of Te Urewera, west of Gisborne. My kuia named me after him (my name Wiremu is a Māori form of William). Te Awhimate's husband, Huatahi NiaNia, whom I called Dad, worked as a shearing, roading and fencing contractor in the hills south of Gisborne, and our whare (house) was in a village called Tiniroto. Te Awhimate guided me in so many ways in my life. Many of the principles I use in my mahi come from her influence. She was recognised as a matekite, someone with spiritual awareness, and became known in our whānau for her healing practice.

Vision

During my childhood I had frequent experiences that years later I realised were out of the ordinary. When I was seven, an incident happened in our whare, a five-bedroom colonial homestead. To get to the wharepaku (toilet) you had to go along a passage at the rear of the house, past the bathroom, around a corner and there it was, next to the washhouse. One evening I came around that bend heading to the toilet, and something stopped me in my tracks. The door to the wharepaku was wide open and there was a man sitting on the toilet.

Seeing him gave me a real fright. Even though I knew he was Māori, he looked quite fair and had gingery hair. He was solidly built and looked about 40. He was wearing a brown knitted pullover and his trousers were around his knees. He was a complete stranger to me. He did not feel threatening, but I found it very strange that he was sitting there on the toilet when he shouldn't be. I backed out and shot down the passage to find my kuia.

When I burst into her bedroom, Nan was lying on her bed. She always worked hard and was resting up after her day's work. She must have been in her 40s at that time but suffered from both asthma and arthritis. The pain in her joints made it uncomfortable for her to stand for long periods. She looked up, ready to growl me for running in the house. Without waiting I shouted, 'E kui! He tangata kei runga i te wharepaku!' (Nan, there is someone on the toilet!). The expression on her face softened and she gave me a kindly look and said, 'Kei te pai boy, kei te pai' (It's okay, boy, it's all right).

I went close to her and stood where she could put her arm around me. She didn't ask me anything about the figure. She knew that there was no one else physically there in the house. No living person was likely to have entered our whare uninvited to use the toilet. She had her own acute awareness of wairua and would have 'seen' what I had seen. Furthermore, she had always known that I was able to see things in the wairua that others couldn't see. She considered it was her job to comfort and awhi (support) me; to help me understand what I was experiencing in the wairua so that I would not lose my mind. She was quite calm, and her demeanour helped me relax a little. 'Kāre e roa ka haere' (He won't be there long. He's just passing through.).

Experiences

This book is about a range of experiences that are less common, such as hearing voices or seeing, feeling or knowing things that may not be shared by others. If no one else can see or hear these things, people who experience them might doubt their own sanity, or others might think they are having psychotic experiences.

Usually, I don't try to consciously analyse the experiences I have; they just happen, and I act on them when that seems appropriate. Also, generally I prefer to view them as a whole. If I hear a voice, most often there is someone I can see who goes with the voice. With those perceptions goes a sense that I can feel them there as well. It's a holistic experience. It hasn't been my habit to break it down and analyse the parts of it. In te ao Māori, it makes more sense to view it as a whole.

However, for the purposes of this book, Allister has encouraged me to analyse some of these experiences: to break them down so others can understand; to look at the nitty-gritty of them to see what we can learn. He tells me that in psychiatry, the content or detail of a person's voices or visions may be considered irrelevant to making sense of their nature or origin. However, for someone such as a clinician who is not matekite, details of how a person describes such experiences may be useful clues. They may reveal cultural indicators that could prompt clinicians to seek advice from a wairua practitioner colleague.

When I think back on this incident with the man on the toilet, I would say that it was mainly a visual experience. You could say it was a vision. I can't recall any smell. I didn't hang around to hear anything. I saw him. I got a fright. But I didn't feel I was in danger of any sort. He didn't move towards me or try to reach out and grab me. These days I would often have a feeling about any person I see in the wairua but I can't recall a feeling emanating from this fella. Perhaps I was too young to make sense of any feeling about him or what his intention was.

That was the first and only time I recall seeing that man. You might ask, could this have been a hallucination? I became acquainted with this term only when I began working in mental health services. After working with youth at risk for many years, in the mid-1990s, I was employed as a cultural worker for mental health services in Gisborne. In 2005 I then moved to Te Whare Mārie in Porirua, where Allister and I began working together.

Wairua

I believe that we are spiritual beings experiencing a human existence. When someone is suffering from seeing or hearing things, it is a common assumption in Western psychiatry that there will be a physical or psychological cause for that. However, in my mahi I look to the spirit first. When someone is hearing voices, seeing visions or having other perceptual experiences, I am curious to assess whether there might be a spiritual cause for this experience. I am looking to the realm of wairua.

The word 'wairua' is often translated into English as meaning 'spiritual', but there is much more to it than that. In order to explain wairua, I refer to the different parts of this kupu (word), 'wa-i-rua'. 'Wa' refers to time and space. The letter 'i' is about the essence of life, and refers to something infinite, beyond time. 'Rua' for me pertains to a receptacle or container. In our ancient schools of learning, 'rua' also means knowledge. There are many levels and types of knowledge. Wairua is the Source of all knowledge that spans time and space. This is why it is possible for some people to see the ancestors of others after they have passed on. The ultimate 'rua' or container of knowledge and healing is my Source. I can do nothing without access to that Source. I often refer to my Source as Io, Te Kaihanga, the Creator, Wairua, the Divine or God.

In order for us as humans to have access to that storehouse of knowledge, we need to be able to receive it, by means beyond the usual senses. I liken this meaning of rua to a television. The signal that is transmitted to the TV cannot be expressed without the receiver that is in the TV. As a matekite, I consider myself to be like that kind of receptacle. The wairua is there and I receive subtle messages or indications of things that have taken place or communications that relate to the nature of wairua.

For me, a spiritual experience is any experience that relates to wairua. It might be a profound moment that goes beyond the physical realm. Other times it may be very simple, for example, sensing a distinct smell or taste, or feeling like someone touched me on the arm when no one is there physically. It could involve a deeper sense of awareness of, or connection to, certain people or places, tīpuna, atua, God or divinity. It can involve a new experience of time. Such an experience might involve intense emotions, communion with nature, dreams or moments of contemplation.

An experience of wairua could happen smack bang out of nowhere. You may have no idea where it came from or why it happened. You may have no sense of control over it. It may feel very positive, or it might feel negative. It is likely to be totally unique to each person and influenced by what they are going through at the time.

We all have different experiences. I may try to interpret that for a person, but I can't know exactly what they were experiencing at the time. I would say that the person who had the experience is the expert on what they went through.

Hallucinations and Wairua

In te ao Māori it is accepted that some people will be able to perceive messages and communications from wairua that others cannot. This is important for how we understand the meaning of the word 'hallucination'. I associate hallucinating with people who may be seeing or hearing things when there is nothing there, perhaps as a result of smoking cannabis or dropping acid or some other substance that can cause such an experience. There are also psychological factors that could cause hallucinations, such as traumatic experiences or physical factors such as a brain injury.

In psychiatry, hallucinations are viewed as significant from a diagnostic perspective and are often used to contribute to a diagnosis of a psychotic illness such as schizophrenia. While I acknowledge this can be justified and useful in some circumstances, over the years people with Māori spiritual experiences have frequently been misdiagnosed as having mental health problems. We have written this book to highlight this distinction and to show how Māori healing and psychiatry working together can help reduce confusion and misdiagnosis and improve the mental health and spiritual care of Māori and perhaps of other Indigenous peoples.

Māori Explanations

There are Māori kupu (words) to describe the gift of being tuned in to wairua experiences. For example, matakite is commonly understood to refer to a person's capacity to experience something beyond the physical realm and may include foresight, the ability to be aware of events before they occur (NiaNia et al., 2017b). Matekite is a related gift that refers to an ability to have insight into or see spirits of those who have passed on or to use spiritual awareness to discern sickness in someone (NiaNia et al., 2017b). I use the following whakatauākī (proverb) to explain this: Mā te kite ka mōhio, mā te mōhio ka kitea he oranga. (By the seeing, one will have knowledge; by that knowledge, one will find an answer.) (NiaNia et al., 2017b).

This proverb highlights not only the capacity for this type of 'vision' but also the potential for healing inherent in such a gift, which is often handed down from generation to generation. I was very fortunate to have my kuia to guide me in the realm of wairua, but young people who are cut off from their elders may have no way to make sense of such voices or visions. An important part of my mahi is explaining wairua to help people figure out these confusing experiences.

While notions of wairua may be unfamiliar to some Western-trained mental health practitioners, I expect spiritual worldviews are common to many Indigenous peoples. I do not consider myself to be an expert when it comes to other Indigenous peoples. I have talked to many people from other Indigenous cultures who have expressed similar ideas, but I still won't assume that I know their culture. Other Indigenous peoples have their own knowledges and stories.

I'm confident that seeing that man on the wharepaku wasn't a hallucination. I believe it was a true perception. I was sure about what I saw. It was as if I was looking at another human being. It was only after my kuia said 'It's all right, he won't be there long' that I realised he was not from this place but rather he was an apparition. At that time, I had no words to describe such a spiritual experience.

Karekau He Rerekē o te Mate o te Ora

My kuia tended not to make a distinction between the living and the dead in her kōrero (conversation) with me. She taught me 'Karekau he rerekē o te mate o te ora': there is no separation between the living and the dead. She maintained that life and death go together, that they are part and parcel of each other and that there is very little difference between this world and the next.

My kuia never used the word 'wairua' with me. She knew I could see things whether they were living or dead. She would say, 'Wire, ka taea e koe te kite ēnei mea' (Wire, you have the ability to see things). Regardless of whether it was a spiritual animal, a spiritual person or any spiritual entity, she would refer to it as if it was present with us. And she would refer to such apparitions by referring to what they were, for example, te tamaiti (the child), te tangata (the person), te hōiho (the horse) or whatever it was. I assume that she spoke in this way in order to normalise my experience, so I would not be afraid.

Kei Tua i te Ārai

At other times my kuia would tell me, 'Kei tua i te ārai' (They are just beyond the veil of death). By referring to a fine barrier or curtain between this world and the next, her explanation helped me understand why I could still perceive them. At other times she would advise me, 'Kei konei tonu' (They are just over here). This was her way of letting me know that there are spirits all around us and that is normal. While they may have left their physical body, they haven't left this physical earth. Even the kōrero at a tangihanga (bereavement ritual) invites our deceased loved ones to stay in relationship with us. For example, we often say, 'Haere haere haere engari hoki wairua mai' (Go but don't leave us: come back spiritually). My encounter with this gentleman in our house was an early occasion when I began to learn that I could feel safe even though a wairua experience might be very vivid and confusing. It often felt to me that my kuia was my guide, almost like my spiritual bodyguard. My response to her reassurance was a feeling that the wairua that I was experiencing was okay. I think she was very comfortable with her own relationship with wairua. Whether that be Io or the holy spirit or any other wairua, she was at ease with that relationship.

Voice Hearing

One example of hearing a voice occurred when I was in my late teens. On that occasion I was driving back from Mahia, about an hour south of Gisborne, in a Standard Ten, an English car from the 1950s, which had very poor brakes. The car was packed with people, loaded up with gear and was pulling a caravan. We had just reached the top of a very steep, narrow winding road. As soon as we started to pick up speed on the other side, someone shouted, 'E Wire!' I jammed on the brakes. As we shuddered slowly to a halt, I shouted angrily, 'What? Are you telling me how to drive?' But no one else had heard it. At that moment, a huge articulated truck came around the corner and bore down on us. If I hadn't slammed the brakes on when I did, I'm certain we all would have been killed as there is no way that truck could have avoided us on such a narrow stretch of road. Either we would have gone over the side or it would have ploughed right into us.

After several incidents where I narrowly avoided death as a result of hearing this same female voice calling 'E Wire!', I consulted my kuia. Her view was that it was very likely to be my adopted mother Nancy, who she was sure had been a kaitiaki (spiritual guardian) for me since Nancy's death when I was one year old.

When I think back on this experience, it's a simple example of hearing a voice. I wasn't aware of seeing anything or having any other feeling, perhaps because I was so busy driving. And the voice shouted, rather than spoke, only two words in my ear: 'E Wire.'

Message

When I hear a voice, I'm not assuming it is meaningless or random. I view it as a form of communication: a source of information and instruction. Generally, I can make sense of what is being communicated by the voice I hear, either then or later. I am interested to understand what the message is.

In the Mahia story, the voice gave me a warning. The message was kia tūpato: watch out! This message was delivered very effectively with one utterance, and it probably saved our lives.

Connection

Another aspect that I am always considering is: what is the relational link or connection? I always assume that if I am getting a message from a voice or other experience that there may be a link through whakapapa (genealogy) or another relationship in the wairua or in my life.

In this story, I couldn't tell straightaway what the relational tie was. It was only years later, after talking to my kuia, that I figured it out. From that conversation I came to understand that I had what is known as a kaitiaki, and I was told that she was my adopted mother, Nancy. After some years I came to trust that voice and to be alert to such warnings.

Later in this book you can read about other kaitiaki experiences through Egan's story in Chapter 5, Tohu's in Chapter 6 and Jake's in Chapter 8.

Te Hua

During a wairua experience such as a voice, I frequently have a clear impression about whether the spiritual entity I'm sensing has a positive intention or not. I can generally tell if it is benevolent or malevolent: if it is there to whakamana me or another person (enhance our mana or spiritual authority) or takahi mana (diminish our mana or spiritual authority); if it is there to support or undermine.

However, apart from that direct feeling, I am also interested to think about te hua, the fruits of this experience. What are the results? What happens in my life or the life of the person affected by it?

When someone asks me, 'Is this a good spirit or a bad spirit?' I think about what impact it is having on this person's life. If they are frothing at the mouth and their head is spinning round and round like a scene from *The Exorcist*, then I would conclude it is probably not a good spirit!

In the case of the voice I heard on the road from Mahia, I can't recall any feeling of good or bad, but with regard to the result, we narrowly avoided a disaster. That tells me it was a good voice, a benevolent entity, and of course I later came to know it as my kaitiaki.

Shared Experience

On the road from Mahia, I had people around me in the car. Despite that, no one else heard the voice I heard. When a person is alone in perceiving a voice or vision, it can lead them to doubt themselves or even their sanity. However, sometimes I've had experiences of hearing things and seeing things in wairua that others have also been able to see and hear.

One example I will never forget happened when I was 19. I was working as a shearer in my father's shearing gang, and we were shearing up at Parikanapa Station, near Tiniroto. They must have had over 3,000 breeding ewes. We were staying in the shearer's quarters about 100 metres up the hill from the shearing shed. That shed would have been more than 60 years old at the time. There were 11 of us there: four of us shearers, four rousies (whose job it was to look after the wool), two pressers and a cook. We would start work at 5 AM and each 'run' would be an hour and 45 minutes. We would knock off for the evening at 5 PM. We would have our dinner about 6 PM and then retire, and some of us would sit around talking and playing cards.

One evening we continued playing cards until midnight, laughing and telling jokes. Suddenly we all stopped. We could distinctly hear the overhead shearing machines come on in the shearing shed down the hill. Listening intently, we could hear laughing, shouting and the sound of sheep bleating, as if they were being herded into the shed. We all stood up to look out the window. It was quite dark outside, but all the lights were on in the shearing shed. We were thinking, 'Who the heck is down there?' None of us were game to go down the hill in the dark to investigate. The noise went on for about half an hour. It sounded just like a normal working shearing shed.

We knew there were no sheep in there. We were on the side of a mountain. This was such a remote spot we knew it was highly unlikely anyone had walked in from the main road. And even if they had, it's a big job to muster sheep into the pens in the shed, let alone in the dark. It would have taken a whole shearing gang working to make it sound like that. When we entered the shed the next morning, there was no sign that anyone had been there. Everything was just as we had left it the day before.

There would have been at least seven of us awake that night who all shared that same experience. It freaked me out at the time, but it was only my fear of the unknown. It didn't actually feel threatening. Since then, I've heard stories from other shearers of similar occurrences that they couldn't explain. Looking back, I think this was a visit from some people who had passed on. Perhaps it was some shearers who had come back to have one last run.

Of course, I can't prove that this was a spiritual thing going on. But what's interesting to me is that all of us shared the experience. We all heard it and saw it. If there was no physical person there causing the ruckus, how do we explain it? According to definitions in psychiatry, if the voices or visions are not based in a tangible external reality, that means they are hallucinations. Was this some kind of mass hallucination phenomena where we were all simultaneously having the same psychotic experience? We hadn't been drinking or using any illicit drugs that night. It was a very long way to the nearest pub. So how can we explain such an experience?

To me, the simplest and most likely explanation comes from wairua. If someone says they are experiencing something but no one else has that experience, and if they are distressed and end up seeing a mental health clinician, they may be diagnosed with a mental illness. If their experience is really from a spiritual origin, and someone else can discern the same experience, then the experience can be verified. A shared experience like this, identified by a Māori healer or other wairua practitioner, could result in developing a dramatically different treatment plan if there is a strong partnership between Māori healing and psychiatry. Jake's chapter gives an example of just such a situation.

If I were to analyse this, I would say that the experience included hearing the sounds of the shearing machines and voices and seeing the lights on in the shearing shed. But not only that: I could feel people down there. I could feel their joy, as if there were men down there who had come back to experience their old shearing life again. The message for all of us was a communication that although they had passed on, they hadn't gone far. They were letting us know that the veil of death is only a thin piece of material. If you have the ability to see beyond that veil, you may see many others who are still in the vicinity.

With regard to the connection, this moment gave us as shearers a link with part of our history. We were the latest generation in a line of people who had done this work, in that woolshed and in that area. The fruit of this experience was the opportunity for a rare demonstration of the mystery of wairua: a startling reminder that the unseen world is very much part of us. While this might have a different meaning for each of us, knowing that life doesn't end just because your body falls could help some of us face death.

Wairua and Māori Healing

The incident at Parikanapa Station was unsettling but ultimately not threatening. However, a contrasting example from my late teenage years was less benign. This story shows how visions associated with wairua can often be accompanied by physical symptoms that closely resemble physical health problems. It also illustrates a Māori healing intervention for what I believe was a wairua problem.

One day when I was working in a rural area of Gisborne as a scrub cutter, a few of us went to the pub after work. By 7 PM or 8 PM we were on our way back to the shearing quarters on a farm in the valley where we were staying. Having had a couple of drinks, I realised that I needed to have a mimi (to urinate). I asked my mate who was driving to pull over at a clear area beside the road. It was dusk and I hopped out of the truck and walked out of sight amongst a few trees and found a discreet place to relieve myself. I then returned to our vehicle, and we continued on our way.

Initially I felt okay, but by about midnight I began to feel sick. It wasn't long before the nausea became intense, and my guts were sore. Not only that, but I was starting to see things. As I lay on my bunk in the dark, I could see what looked like dark human faces and figures coming straight at my eyes. They appeared to be human, but the shadowy images would break up into fragments just as they reached my face. They felt unfriendly, as if I was being harassed, but they were inaudible. There was no let-up; they were coming in a continuous stream. Soon I felt overwhelmed and started vomiting and sweating like I had a fever.

These experiences went on all night: by morning, I was exhausted. My boss came to see me in bed and told me he had arranged to take me back into town to drop me off with my whānau. When I got there, my whānau members planned to take me to a doctor but when they phoned my kuia she told them to taihoa (wait) while she arranged for someone to see me. Puriri, an old tohunga (Māori healer) in our whānau, arrived at the house to see me in the early afternoon.

I was lying in bed when Puriri knocked quietly and entered my room. The sound of his footsteps on the bare boards reverberated as he walked into the centre of the room and looked at me lying there. He must have been almost 80 and had a striking presence enhanced by his gabardine coat and fedora hat. For quite a while he remained silent. I just lay there looking up at him. He had a kindly face and as we were related, I had known him for some time. I knew he was a man of few words, but I felt relieved that he was there with me. Even though I expected to have to see a doctor, it was common in our whānau to see a tohunga if someone suspected a wairua problem. I knew my kuia had called him and felt confident he could help me. After some time, he spoke: 'I know what's wrong, boy.'

I waited to see what else he had to say. In the meantime, he reached into his jacket pocket and pulled out a well-worn penny. He walked over, sat down on the side of my bed and gestured for me to lie on my back. He laid the penny on my bare chest, over my sternum. After leaving it there for a few moments, he grasped it in his large fingers and rubbed it up and down the centre of my chest a few times while reciting a karakia (prayer) under his breath. Then he wrapped the coin in a white handkerchief and carefully put it back in the top pocket of his gabardine jacket.

He then stood up and looked at me for a moment. 'You've done something, eh boy?'

Puriri seemed to know I was reaping the consequences for doing something to desecrate a person or place. I couldn't think of anything I'd done, so I had no idea what to make of his mysterious intervention. However, by the following day it dawned on me that there was a link between my action at the side of the road the evening before and being unwell. I can now see that the job of my koroua (elder) in this situation was to 'take it off me'. Puriri made a spiritual exchange for my misdemeanour, like a spiritual payment for what I had done. I believe he would have buried that coin afterwards so that no one else could use it. This is an example of the concept of utu. Utu is about reciprocity. It refers to the cost of something, like a principle of exchange. If I have committed a negative deed, there is a cost resulting from that, perhaps in the physical realm, or it could be in the spiritual realm. If I understand that and can make amends for my misdeed, then the matter can be resolved.

After he left, I lay in bed for a few more hours. There were no more visions, my fever abated, and my nausea quickly settled. By nightfall I was feeling better, and by the following morning I had made a full recovery.

Two days later, a friend and I returned to that spot. It was overgrown but we could tell it was a gravesite. The gate was open, and in the twilight, I hadn't noticed where I was. There was a mound there but no gravestone or other marker. I later learned that in this area there were unmarked graves relating to events such as the 1869 massacre at Ngātapa, when Crown forces executed at least 120 of Te Kooti Arikirangi's followers, and the 1918 flu pandemic (Belich, 1996). Te Kooti was a Māori prophet and guerilla leader and had his own experiences of visions and voices, which we will return to in Chapter 2.

In relieving myself, I had unintentionally desecrated someone's grave. This was a violation of tapu, something sacred or forbidden. If I believe there is no separation between the living and the dead, I can tread on someone's mana, their spiritual authority, even if they are dead, and that may have consequences. In my Māori worldview, it is quite possible that a spiritual transgression can result in a physical or mental health problem. In te ao Māori, there is no separation between the spiritual and the physical or mental. We are whole beings, so any aspect of our tinana (physical side), hinengaro (psychological side) or wairua can be affected by a spiritual problem.

A doctor might ask if my symptoms could have been caused by a gastro bug. However, when that happened to me in the past, I didn't see faces or feel like I was being harassed. From my perspective, this was a spiritual problem manifesting as a mixture of physical, mental and spiritual feelings and perceptions.

This experience was a lesson in the need to respect the living and the dead: to take great care not to desecrate tapu places that have been set aside for people to rest in peace. A further point from this story is that if there is a spiritual problem, it follows in te ao Māori that there could be a spiritual resolution. In this book, we are addressing the matter of negative perceptual experiences and whether they might be hallucinations or spiritual experiences. My encounter with Puriri was a story of Māori healing illustrating how such experiences can be addressed. While Puriri's methods might be puzzling from a Western perspective, the outcome for me was evidence that his intervention worked. At the time I didn't understand why it worked, but I now know that he was accessing Māori knowledge that had been passed down to him. While Māori knowledge informs one side of the partnership between Allister and me, the other side relates to Western medical and psychological know-how.

Allister

Early Influences

I grew up in Christchurch, in New Zealand's South Island, and have Irish and English ancestors who immigrated to the Canterbury area in the late 1800s. Growing up in a church community with a social justice ethos but with little exposure to Māori and Pacific cultural values and beliefs, I was curious to learn more. I stayed in the South Island to study medicine in Dunedin, then moved to Hawke's Bay on the east coast of the North Island for my first job as a junior doctor. I was introduced to Māori and Pacific cultural life through patients and friends I met there.

During this time, in the late 1980s, New Zealand's Ministry of Health was grappling with its obligations under the Treaty of Waitangi, the country's founding document. Signed in 1840, the treaty is an agreement between the British Crown and about 540 Māori rangatira (chiefs).

It was well known that most Māori individuals and families refused to attend mental health services unless they were compelled to. For years, Māori health leaders had been advocating for services for Māori, run by Māori and staffed by Māori. In the late 1980s the first kaupapa Māori (Māori-centred) mental health unit was set up near Hamilton, in the Waikato region of the central North Island, at Tokanui Psychiatric Hospital.

Māori Rōpū

Around the same time, in Porirua Hospital, another large mental hospital further south, Māori nurses and other Māori staff had been campaigning to open a Māori unit. The Māori Rōpū, as this group was called, invited kaumātua (elders) from Tokanui to visit, to hear about the developments in the Waikato. Pikau Te Rangi Arthur, who was employed as a carpenter around the hospital, was also a senior kaumātua for Ngāti Toa Rangatira, the local iwi (tribe). The iwi recommended him for the role of kaumātua to the Māori Rōpū. Shortly after, Ani Sweet was appointed as the kuia kaumātua (female elder). Other leaders included Māori cooks who would prepare kai (food) such as rēwena bread (sourdough potato bread) and boil up (a traditional Māori stew) to manaaki (support) Māori patients and Māori events at Porirua Hospital.

As part of the group's campaign, a white Toyota hatchback packed with Māori Rōpū leaders set off on a road trip to see how mental health units around the North Island were addressing Māori mental health needs. Some of the original waiata (songs) that are now part of the identity of our Māori mental health service were first rehearsed during that trip.

The Māori Rōpū campaign for a Māori mental health service was successful, and the new service opened in 1990. The service centred around a marae (Māori meeting house) called Te Whare Mārie, which translates into English as 'the house of peace'. This name was bestowed upon the marae by Pikau. The unit initially functioned as a day programme and soon expanded into a full kaupapa Māori outpatient mental health service.

My Experience at Te Whare Mārie

I spent a year working at Te Whare Mārie as a psychiatry trainee in the mid to late 1990s. The Māori cultural context of the service was poles apart from my white, middle-class, Protestant upbringing.

Te Whare Mārie's surroundings made an immediate impact on me. It was at the end of a bush-clad driveway, with a large ponga (tree fern) by the front door. While the peeling red paint on the corrugated iron roof and the creamy yellow weatherboards gave the impression of a farmhouse, Te Whare Mārie had previously been a villa housing elderly patients in the

Porirua Hospital complex. For many, a psychiatric admission to this mental hospital had been a life sentence.

The whare kitchen was often a hub of activity, with staff crowding around the large wooden table clasping hot drinks or eating cereal or toast after the morning hui (meeting). There were invariably noisy conversations to negotiate car availability and to plan community visits and appointments. Around us were relics from the hospital's heyday: a large vintage industrial gas stove, still in service for marae catering, alongside a disused food steamer. Outside the whare, horses grazed on the grassy hillside.

A large living area at one end of the villa had been turned into a marae. From the lawn outside, manuhiri (visitors) would approach the door of the marae during a pōwhiri (ceremonial welcome) for new tāngata whaiora (literally, seekers of wellbeing), whānau and staff. The marae was the site of many significant cultural and clinical activities at Te Whare Mārie, including morning hui, pōwhiri, poroaki (ceremonial farewells) and multidisciplinary team meetings.

As kaumātua, Pikau and Ani guided matters on the marae, ensuring values of manaaki (hospitality) and Ngāti Toa Rangatira tikanga (protocol) were adhered to. The presence of Māori elders at this service differed from any other mental health service I had known in my training.

As well as the formal marae ceremonies, Māori practices such as commencing and finishing meetings with karakia were in sharp contrast to the secular approaches of all the mainstream mental health services I had previously worked in. Mihimihi, where staff and whaiora would introduce themselves with detailed accounts of their tribal connections and ancestry, and where potential connections were celebrated rather than assiduously avoided, were new to me; I'd had no exposure to any of these cultural approaches in my upbringing. There were also differences in the ways people related to each other that I found disquieting. In the morning kitchen scene at Te Whare Mārie, there were multiple conversations all tumbling over each other. If I had waited politely until there was a break in the flurry of kōrero to speak, as I was accustomed to doing in my family of origin, I would never have got a word in.

The Family Centre

My earlier experience in a volunteer placement gave me some experience to bring to Te Whare Mārie. A few years earlier I'd had the privilege of spending a year at The Family Centre, an Anglican social services agency in Lower Hutt, in the Wellington region of the North Island. The Family Centre specialised in family therapy, community work and social policy research. It was one of the first agencies in Aotearoa to adopt a three tikanga approach in which Māori, Samoan and Pākehā sections operated in parallel with one another.

This agency incorporated practices of accountability in order to address historical injustice (Waldegrave et al., 2003). In matters of culture and social justice, the Pākehā section was considered accountable to the Māori and Samoan sections. In matters relating to gender, the male caucus was considered accountable to the female caucus. The idea behind this arrangement was that groups that have been treated unjustly are in the best position to judge if an injustice has been properly addressed. Through the guidance and teaching of Warihi Campbell, Flora Tuhaka, Taimalieutu Kiwi Tamasese and Charles Waldegrave I became acquainted first-hand with Māori and Samoan cultural processes and practices of which I had no prior experience in my upbringing or previous training.

Spirituality was a core value as part of the Family Centre's social justice approach and tikanga. While there had been little mention of the significance of wairua in my undergraduate medical training, at the Family Centre, I became much more aware of the centrality of spirituality to my Māori and Samoan colleagues and how this could be addressed in therapeutic work with families. At the Family Centre, relationships were considered to be at the heart of their shared understandings of spirituality. They explained spirituality in terms of four key relationships: those between people and their environment; those between 'people and other people in terms of love and justice'; those between people and their ancestors or heritage; and those between people and the 'numinous'. They defined the numinous as referring to that which is 'beyond, transcendent, or what some people call God' (Waldegrave et al., 2003, p. 165). These understandings of spirituality made an impact on me because they were very different to what I grew up with. I don't recall giving any thought to defining spirituality in my younger years, but any implicit assumptions I had would have been more focused on individual experience, without reference to the environment or ancestors.

Given that Wiremu has defined wairua in this chapter and this book is about both Māori healing and psychiatry perspectives, here is a definition of spirituality from a modern textbook on spirituality and psychiatry:

> Spirituality is a … dimension of human experience arising both within the inner subjective awareness of individuals and within communities, social groups and traditions. It may be experienced as relationship with that which is intimately 'inner', immanent and personal, within the self and others, and/or as relationship with that which is wholly 'other', transcendent and beyond the self. It is experienced as being of fundamental or ultimate importance and is thus concerned with matters of meaning and purpose in life, truth, and values.
>
> (Cook et al., 2009)

As with the Family Centre definition, this definition of spirituality is much broader than just referring to religion. It is also expressed in terms of relationship, but without specific reference to environment or ancestors which are considered so significant in Māori and Pacific cultural settings. The following account illustrates a further point of contrast.

It was at the Family Centre that I first heard a story about Warihi being asked by a psychiatrist to see two tormented prison inmates. They were under assessment for possible psychosis due to their experience of seeing a troubling figure in their cell who was not apparent to other people (Waldegrave et al., 2003). However, this disturbing shared experience resolved rapidly after Warihi entered their cell and blessed them and the cell with karakia and holy water. This story intrigued me because it raised the possibility there could be a Māori explanation for some mysterious and compelling perceptual experiences, and that this could be effectively addressed with a Māori cultural and spiritual solution.

There were kaimahi (workers) at Te Whare Mārie who would have been aware of the significance of Māori cultural and spiritual experiences, but I wasn't attuned to such matters. Instead, I was engrossed in learning my trade as a psychiatrist and absorbing the teachings that had been handed down to me in our professional texts. The task was to memorise and apply the established definitions of types of hallucinations and other psychiatric symptoms rather than question their relevance for the experiences of some of the people we were meeting.

Hallucinations and Psychiatry

According to one commonly used definition at that time, a hallucination was 'a sensory perception that has the compelling sense of reality of a true perception but that occurs without external stimulation of the relevant sensory organ' (American Psychiatric Association, 1994).

The tacit assumption in scientific medical discourse was that if a visual experience was not visible or an auditory experience was not audible to the clinician or others present, then by definition there was 'no external stimulation' and the experience therefore constituted a hallucination. There was little room in such medical teaching for the possibility that there might be subtle spiritual or cultural awareness of some entity in the spiritual realm that represented a true perception – or that such a perception could be shared by members of a culture who were attuned to such experiences.

Non-pathological Hallucinations

In my training, psychiatry acknowledged that some hallucinatory experiences could be non-pathological, such as the hallucinatory experiences many people report in the moments before falling asleep or while waking up. It was also well known that recently bereaved people often reported seeing a deceased loved one. This visual hallucination was considered to be non-pathological and somehow caused by an acute grief reaction. Again, the tacit assumption was that this experience was not a true perception of the spirit of the deceased person, but a hallucinated product of the mind of the grieving person.

Other examples of non-pathological hallucinations I learnt about included the visual disturbances experienced by people with marked visual impairment known as Charles Bonnet syndrome. More often associated with elderly people, these visual disturbances were said to include perceiving quite complex visual images such as animals, people and detailed landscapes, houses or other structures, which could be still or moving (Sims, 1995). These experiences were usually present in the absence of any other brain abnormality or other signs of a significant mental health problem.

Auditory and Visual Hallucinations

We were taught that while auditory or verbal hallucinations were commonly associated with major psychotic disorders such as schizophrenia or mood states such as mania or severe depression, visual hallucinations were much less common in such mental health disorders and could indicate the presence of an organic brain problem. One example frequently cited was visual hallucinations associated with acute withdrawal for someone addicted to alcohol. Such experiences were one symptom of a particular type of delirium known as delirium tremens or 'the DTs'. A memorable example described in the textbooks was that of Lilliputian hallucinations in which the sufferer 'sees' tiny creatures or people, associated with strong feelings such as terror (Sims, 1995). Other abnormal perceptions such as those relating to the sense of smell, known as olfactory hallucinations, were also considered to indicate possible brain problems such as seizures in specified parts of the brain, particularly the temporal lobes.

While training and working in hospitals as junior doctors, all medical practitioners will have seen situations where people who are medically unwell experience the sudden onset of disturbing perceptual experiences such as voices or visions. These experiences are considered to be the direct result of the illness on that person's brain. This pattern of symptoms, also a form of acute delirium, can often be effectively and promptly addressed by appropriate treatment of the medical condition and sometimes with antipsychotic medications used to treat major psychotic illnesses. After seeing such an obvious link between a physical cause for hallucinations and immediate benefit from a medication considered to block dopamine receptors in the brain, I found the idea that hallucinations were caused by a physical or chemical problem in the brain very compelling. It fitted very well with what I already understood.

At the same time, while we were encouraged to consider cultural perspectives as part of a bio-psycho-social approach to understanding our patient's predicaments, there was little guidance on how to identify whether a Māori patient was having a Māori cultural experience as opposed to a hallucination. My Scottish psychiatrist supervisor at Te Whare Mārie did mention that she believed that some Māori patients' experiences could have been cultural rather than psychiatric. In addition, textbooks described a range of 'culture-bound syndromes' from other parts of the world and recommended consulting cultural experts to help distinguish a delusion[1] from an accepted cultural belief. However, I don't recall any other detailed advice about how to distinguish between Māori or other cultural experiences and psychotic symptoms in teaching sessions I attended as a trainee psychiatrist in the mid-to-late1990s.

Since then, there have been developments in psychiatric research and theory relating to auditory, visual and other hallucinations, as well as in the burgeoning fields of cultural psychiatry and critical psychiatry. In addition, there have been strong contributions from the Hearing Voices movement and other consumer commentators. We will examine some of these developments in more detail in Chapters 4 and 5.

After completing my training in psychiatry in Wellington and having more training in child and adolescent psychiatry in Lower Hutt and Melbourne, Australia, I returned to New Zealand and started working at Te Whare Mārie in 2005 as a consultant child and adolescent psychiatrist. A month later, Wiremu joined the service as a cultural therapist. We got on well from the outset, but he was silent about the nature of his cultural therapy work and it was several years before I became curious about his ideas and therapeutic approaches.

Wiremu and Caleb

One of the first times I had an opportunity to question Wiremu about his ideas and practice related to a 17-year-old man called Caleb who came to our service following an unusual and terrifying experience. While walking out his front door on his way to school, Caleb was confronted by a Māori man shouting at him. He saw the head and upper torso of this life-size and threatening figure next to his letterbox, brandishing a taiaha (long wooden Māori weapon). Caleb had Māori on one side of his family and Cook Island Māori on the other and had grown up with his Cook Island Māori family. However, he was sure this warrior-like figure was shouting at him in te reo

Māori (the Māori language). This story has been described in detail in our first book (NiaNia et al., 2017).

I was perplexed by this young person's disturbing experience. I was struck by the way he described his visual and auditory experience as synchronised, for example with the figure's mouth appearing to move in time with the words he was shouting. In contrast, auditory hallucinations accompanying psychotic illness are often described as emanating from thin air. His detailed description impressed me as having distinctly cultural features, especially when Caleb's te reo Māori teacher arranged for him to see a tohunga at school after he reluctantly told her about his experiences. When this Māori elder recited a karakia while blessing Caleb by tossing handfuls of water over him, the experiences immediately ceased. This didn't make sense to me from a psychiatric point of view. If it was a hallucination, why would it disappear just like that?

I had my first appointment with Caleb after Wiremu had met with him. After hearing his story, I was curious to ask Wiremu what he thought was going on. His first response took me by surprise. Wiremu told me that as soon as he heard Caleb's account, he was convinced this young man had, through some action, inadvertently brought the situation about. One of his first questions to Caleb was to ask what he had picked up. As a psychiatrist, nothing in my paradigm would have led me to ask that question.

Wiremu's enquiry went something like this: 'Well, it looks to me like something's happened here, or you have done something or picked something up. Can you tell me if you picked anything up?' Caleb responded, 'A couple of weeks ago I found this piece of pounamu (a precious greenstone pendant) on the road and I picked it up and put it around my neck because it was a nice-looking piece of pounamu.' And Wiremu's response was, 'That's the answer. That is the reason that you have had this experience. Let's see if we can find an appropriate way to resolve this.'

Mauri, Tapu and Mana

Wiremu then told me about three Māori concepts that I was only dimly aware of: mauri, tapu and mana (NiaNia et al., 2017b). Wiremu assured me that these words held the key to understanding Caleb's predicament. He described mauri as a person's life force, which could become attached to something like a piece of pounamu, over time, if it was worn close to their skin. He described tapu as something sacred or forbidden and said that by picking up someone else's pounamu pendant and wearing it, Caleb had inadvertently breached a tapu. As a result of this breach, it was likely that the ancestors of the person who had lost the pounamu had become angry. Wiremu told me he was sure Caleb's vision and the shouting that he heard in synchrony with this vision were a Māori cultural or spiritual experience that had a logical cultural cause and could be addressed with an appropriate cultural solution.

So here was a vivid example for me of a vision and an associated voice that were highly disturbing for a young person. From my psychiatrist's perspective, Caleb's experience fitted the definition of visual hallucinations with associated auditory hallucinations. However, there was no evidence of any other psychotic symptoms, such as delusions or formal thought disorder. Caleb didn't report recent drug use or a medical condition that might have been a possible cause of a psychotic experience such as hallucinations. This apparent hallucinatory experience didn't fit neatly into an established psychiatric diagnostic category.

There was also evidence supporting Wiremu's explanation. Caleb's disturbing experiences ended as soon as he was blessed by the tohunga. Caleb described hearing a voice shouting at him in what he recognised as te reo Māori but that included unfamiliar words and phrases. Caleb's vision included features that Wiremu identified as being typical of a Māori cultural experience, including the nature of the challenge and the appearance and clothing of the figure, who had a facial tattoo. Finally, while Caleb found his experience totally unexpected and shocking, Wiremu was able to provide a coherent Māori explanation that accounted for the appearance of this figure, at this time in Caleb's life, based on Māori concepts. After hearing this explanation, Caleb told me that it made sense to him. He felt reassured that his experience was understandable from a Māori point of view, and that Wiremu could help him deal with it.

Early Understanding

Wiremu's explanation enabled me to start to understand the logic of approaching Caleb's predicament from a Māori perspective, even though it was unfamiliar to me. Wiremu was able to teach me in a very accessible way: 'If you want to understand Caleb's experience, you can think of it as a spiritual germ that this young person picked up.' Later, I realised Wiremu had used a medical metaphor to help me as a doctor to understand a Māori spiritual concept.

Furthermore, Wiremu was strongly focused on assisting Caleb to become aware of the nature of his problem. He was sure gaining more understanding would ease Caleb's fear. For some weeks after his experiences ended, following the intervention of the tohunga, Caleb continued to have panic attacks. Wiremu focused on illuminating the Māori reasons for the experience for Caleb and carrying out the necessary Māori solution, which was to dispose of the pounamu appropriately. Afterwards, Caleb's panic episodes gradually settled.

Partnership

By the time of Wiremu's departure from Te Whare Mārie in 2010, we had been seeing young people and their families together for several years and had many discussions about our different Māori and psychiatry perspectives. At that point Wiremu suggested that we write a book together. That first book took seven years to reach publication. Wiremu was very motivated to give mental health clinicians an opportunity to read about Māori understandings of unusual perceptual experiences. I was interested in the way Wiremu was able to teach me about his experience of wairua and his Māori world views. I was keen for other clinicians to be able to read Wiremu's explanations for puzzling experiences Māori and Pacific young people were having that didn't fit neatly into the usual psychological or psychiatric categories.

During our many discussions I noticed that Wiremu had no problem with me holding firmly to my psychiatry points of view. I'm sure he could see that I was sceptical about some of his views about wairua, and he would often arrange for me to follow up something he had noticed with a family in order that I could verify it for myself. I realised we could work together effectively even if we didn't share the same beliefs about some things. I observed that he was very respectful of whatever spiritual beliefs a family might have and while generous in sharing his explanations, he was very careful not to impose his ideas about spirituality on any families we met.

Wiremu was able to provide explanations about wairua and spiritual problems that made sense to me, as a Pākehā doctor unfamiliar with te ao Māori. This helped considerably in my understanding of these territories of experience that I found so unfamiliar and mysterious. It was later pointed out to me that while it was very obliging of Wiremu to illuminate these matters for me, the validity of these Māori constructs does not depend on Pākehā appraisal. Wiremu's Māori paradigms are not required to be 'coherent' from a Western perspective.

Matekite and Psychiatry

I noticed that many of the young people and families Wiremu and I met together with found it very easy to understand and accept Wiremu's Māori explanations for what they were going through. They resonated immediately. When Wiremu identified that a young person was having spiritual experiences that might be disturbing, he would say they had a spiritual gift that may have been passed down in their family. I'd never read about this idea in any psychiatric textbook, yet it was relevant to my work at Te Whare Mārie. The young people he was referring to frequently described seeing human-looking figures that others couldn't see, or hearing voices guiding them or harassing them, or knowing things they couldn't have been expected to know through their usual senses. They had intense intuitive feelings about people or places that were not evident to others and that strongly influenced their behaviour.

When I asked these young people and their families for more detail, I discovered that they had often been having experiences like this for many years, even going back to their early childhood. After more inquiries, it was usually possible to find other family members who had similar experiences. These abilities could be traced back to aunties, uncles, grandparents and other family members.

You can read about young people with such experiences in later chapters, including Jake in Chapter 8. Wiremu explained that such matekite experiences are commonly accepted in Māori thinking. Language, knowledge systems and elders are there to guide and support young people with these experiences. He said it was a major problem for Māori who are tuned in to spiritual experiences to encounter psychiatrists and others in the mental health field with no knowledge of such matters. This was why Wiremu was keen for us to write a second book, this time focused on voices and visions from both Māori healing and psychiatric points of view. A further purpose for me has been to examine the question of whether there is intellectual space in psychiatry to include Māori and other spiritual perspectives in our thinking about mental health and the problems for which people seek our assistance.

Wiremu

How We Wrote This Book

This book has come about through many conversations between Allister and me about people we have met and how to explain their unusual experiences so that others may understand. From audio-recordings of all that kōrero, Allister transcribed and edited the text and David Epston, our colleague and friend, helped edit it to make it more readable, asking many probing questions and providing regular encouragement. Allister and I have often sat together reviewing and revising drafts of each chapter.

We audio-recorded some sessions, with the permission of the families, and some kōrero is quoted directly so you can see exactly what was said. But it's not just about what Allister and I think. We have invited other participants from each story to give their account: to describe in their own words the detail of their unusual experiences and their own views about wairua and the resolution of their suffering. We think their words bring these stories to life, and we are very grateful for their generosity in sharing their kōrero about some of the most vulnerable moments in their lives.

Tātaihono

Allister and I have now been working together for 18 years. Since I left Te Whare Mārie, we have continued to see families together from time to time, to teach, to present workshops and to write together. During this time, Allister and I have continued to develop our model of collaboration. The name I gave to that is Tātaihono. Tātaihono is about bringing the Māori and Pākehā elements together and binding them in such a way that the mana of each paradigm is enhanced. This approach requires mutual trust and transparency, understanding, respect and lots of kōrero. We have spent many hours over the years enquiring about each other's worldviews. We have had to find a way to kōrero about the history between our cultures, and the impact of colonisation on the marginalisation of Māori worldviews. We have had to develop a shared tikanga for sessions when we are working together. We have learnt that neither of us has to compromise the important values that underpin our Māori and professional psychiatric knowledge systems in order for whānau to benefit from this partnership. We have found that the different knowledge streams can complement each other, and that whānau we work with want to have access to both.

In Chapter 2, I explain Māori meanings of seeing visions and hearing voices as they were handed down to me and as I have come to understand them from other sources. Too often Indigenous perspectives have been sidelined, silenced or absent from this kōrero. I show how knowledge about te ao wairua (the spiritual realm) can inform our understanding of voices and visions.

In Chapter 3, Allister and I delve into European examples of people who experienced voices and visions in the past.

In Chapter 4, Allister details perspectives from psychiatry over the years and I offer comments in response.

In Chapter 5, our colleague Egan Bidois shares his experiences and insights into wairua and other voices and visions that severely affected him as a young man. He describes his treatment in a psychiatric hospital in the early 1990s and discusses how he learned to live with these experiences.

Chapters 6 to 8 consist of stories that have been gifted by people Allister and I worked with, so we can all learn more about wairua and healing. Tohu's story in Chapter 6 illustrates how an unusual perceptual experience can be used for healing. In Chapter 7, Grace's story describes her distressing experiences of a voice and visions and how she and her whānau were able to address them. It gives a detailed account of the family healing session that Allister and I had with Grace and her family, to illustrate our partnership in action. Jake's narrative in Chapter 8 describes his experiences of voices and visions and his interactions with Allister and me after he was referred to Te Whare Mārie. We document his progress over the subsequent ten years and his understandings of his experiences and their meaning in his life.

In Chapter 9, I provide a detailed account of my approach to addressing wairua in my mahi.

Finally, in Chapter 10, Allister outlines approaches to distinguishing wairua from hallucinations in psychiatric practice, and I offer my commentary in response. We finish with an update on Caleb's story, more than a decade after I first met him, as he recounts further experiences of voices and visions and their meaning in his life.

Notes

1 Delusions are defined in psychiatry as fixed false beliefs not consistent with the person's cultural background and not amenable to reason. In the rest of this book, we will refer to a brief version of this definition, 'fixed false beliefs' for those readers unfamiliar with this term.

2 Tirohanga

Wiremu NiaNia and Allister Bush

Wiremu

In this chapter, we will look at a variety of meanings given to experiences of hearing voices and seeing visions in te ao Māori (the Māori world). 'Tiro' means to observe or examine, and 'tirohanga' in this context is about looking into what our kōrero (explanation) has been about these matters. It is about seeking what is on the other side of ngā kūaha – the doorways of understanding we as a people have – that help us make sense of these less common perceptual experiences.

We will look at examples from pūrākau (Māori narratives), ngā poropiti (Māori prophets), everyday experiences, Māori healing and Māori literature. I hope these stories shed light on various ways wairua (spiritual) experiences might be perceived, to assist us in making sense of voices and visions in relation to mental wellbeing. If hallucinations, as Allister was taught, are perceptions that have no external stimulus, then that means to me there is no cause for that experience outside of the person. Wairua experiences for me are not hallucinations. When I see someone's ancestor there in the room with us, I believe that there is an external spiritual presence that explains my experience. For example, in Chapter 8, Jake and I both perceive the same three entities in the room with us. The fact that Allister didn't notice them there doesn't mean they were hallucinations.

In Western academic writing, credibility is usually given to written sources from reputable texts or journals. However, in te ao Māori, the most tapu or sacred knowledge has always been passed down orally. This creates a dilemma for me. Much important kōrero about the meaning of experiences such as hearing voices and seeing visions may not have been written down. As you will see, the nature of the experiences documented by these authors reflects the significance these experiences had for them at the time. Everyday experiences, like someone seeing their deceased kuia (female elder) before their eyes, would have been considered so ordinary that there was no point writing about it.

DOI: 10.4324/9781003187042-2

When I reflect on the word 'kūaha', as well as referring to an opening or doorway, it can be split into 'ku' and 'aha'. The syllable 'ku' can refer to something belonging to me, and 'aha' is about my intent. This chapter is about what has been documented about voices and visions in Māori writing. Nevertheless, I have chosen to cross the threshold of some entranceways and not others. This kōrero reflects my own personal search for what can help us understand perceptions relating to wairua. Others may see things very differently.

Ngā Taonga Tuku Iho

My starting point for this kōrero is ngā taonga tuku iho – knowledge handed down to us from our ancestors. For me that begins with my earliest education at the feet of my kuia, Te Awhimate. This was well before the days of TV. After dinner, when the chickens and pigs were fed and the dishes done, we would gather around her in front of the fire. I remember the smell of mānuka logs burning in the grate: my kuia leaning forward on her comfy couch with eyes sparkling and her gaze seeking our attention; us kids sitting cross-legged on our rimu timber floor, staring up at her, keenly anticipating the evening's entertainment. All her kōrero was in te reo (the Māori language). Her favourite tales ranged from the escapades of atua (deities) and ancestors to narratives of wairua (spirituality), creation and divinity. My kuia spoke of people who could see and hear things in wairua, and those who had dreams foretelling the future. She had a particular predilection for things that go bump in the night.

In te ao Māori the origin of perception is found in our creation narratives. According to my kuia, the beginning of everything was our creator, Io. Out of Io came Te Kore, which is often translated as 'the void'. In this state, there was no time, and nothing to perceive, but at the same time infinite potential. She explained that Te Kore teaches us that even if you start from nothing, if you follow the wairua and work at it, if you believe, many things are possible.

Next came Te Pō, a stage of impenetrable darkness. Nothing could be seen, but now there was the potential for other senses, like touch and the perception of sound. We have names for that such as Te Pō-tē-kitea, the night in which nothing could be seen, and Te Pō-whāwhā, the darkness in which something could be touched. These names imply the potential for tactile and sound perception and for sensing light even if you have never known it before.

Finally, after many aeons, came the various stages of Te Ao – the world of light.

One of our most well-known pūrākau or creation narratives recounts the story of Papatūānuku, Mother Earth, and Ranginui (Rangi), the Sky Father, who were entwined in such a tight embrace that no light could reach their many children squashed between their bodies. Eventually these atua siblings became frustrated with their confinement.

Uepoto

Uepoto was the first sibling to perceive light. Being curious and restless, he was exploring the outer edges of the torso of Papatūānuku one day when he saw something twinkle. Given he had never known anything but blackness, he rubbed his eyes, wondering, 'What the heck was that?' Then he saw it again: hīnātore – a distinct glimmer of light. A luminescence that glowed softly but steadily in the darkness. Some say he had spotted the radiance of a glow worm in the kēkē, the hollow part of his mother's armpit.

When Uepoto found his way back to where his siblings were, despite his confusion he was itching to let the others know about it. He blurted out, 'Guess what I saw!' However, not one of them believed him. This raises an important matter about the nature of perception. What we perceive is inherently private. Even if we are sitting together looking at the same vista, no one else can tell exactly what we are seeing or hearing unless we communicate our experience. This is much more so for subtle perceptions and especially for wairua experiences. If others have never known anything similar to the experience you are having, naturally they may not believe you. This could lead you to doubt your experience or even seriously question your own sanity.

It was much later when Uepoto's brother, Tāne, first saw light for himself. When he reported this back to the other siblings, they began to take the idea seriously. They held a hui or meeting in which there was a heated debate about whether to separate their parents to relieve the darkness and severe restriction of their circumstances. Eventually it was Tāne who succeeded in forcing Rangi and Papa apart, and they were delivered into Te Ao Mārama – the world of light.

Kahupō

Rūaumoko, the youngest sibling, was the most severely affected by the separation of his parents. At this time, he was in his mother's womb. While the other atua had all been freed by Tāne's actions, Rūaumoko remained surrounded by his waikahu, his amniotic fluid, and surrounded in darkness inside Papatūānuku. While for most unborn babies, the womb must be warm and comforting, Rūaumoko was unable to be born and began to find his confinement intolerable. Over a long time, he felt increasingly pōuri (sad), alienated, lonely and confused. He was in a state of kahupō. Kahu refers to a cloak and you could say he was cloaked in darkness, a state of vulnerability, of not knowing. A similar concept, whaiao, refers to a state of not seeing, both physically and metaphorically – you can't see your future; you can't see where you are or where you are going. You can't see te ara – the pathway forward.

As Rūaumoko's frustration mounted, eruptions reverberated deep within Papatūānuku – expressions of Rūaumoko's distress and violent anger. Of course, we now know Rūaumoko as the atua of earthquakes and volcanoes. But for me, his state of kahupō can help us understand the experiences of people who hear troubling voices or see disturbing visions and have no way to make sense of them. Such experiences are frequently isolating and traumatic. They may shake a person's foundations and lead to them doubting anything they thought they knew about themselves. In this state of alienation, some may contemplate suicide. Whakamomori refers to taking one's own life and captures the sense of confusion, grief, trauma or desperation that may lead someone to that point.

To tell someone they are experiencing an auditory hallucination or psychosis may be well intentioned but, to my mind, this is a very thin kōrero. It may not help them fathom what is going on. There is a saying, 'Kei hea te matū o te kōrero?' which means 'Where is the substance of the kōrero? Where is the richness of what has been said?' Matū refers to the gist, the essence of the kōrero. What is worthwhile listening to? When there is no matū, there is little to sustain the listener. A diagnostic label may offer very few handholds or footholds to help someone climb out of the hole they find themselves in. Mātauranga Māori or Māori knowledge, through the stories of our ancestors, provides many more rich and familiar metaphors and understandings that our people can grasp hold of in their most desperate moments. Kahupō implies that the veil of darkness can be lifted. Resolution is about bringing a light of understanding to that situation to address the confusion and fear. Māori healing offers a relational space in which such a kōrero could take place. We will look at a few examples of Māori healing later in this chapter.

Hine-pūkohu-rangi and Voice Hearing

My kuia told us that the people from our iwi (tribe), Ngāi Tūhoe, are descended from an ancient atua called Hine-pūkohu-rangi. She is known as the goddess of the mist, and this is one reason why Tūhoe are referred to as 'children of the mist'. Hine-pūkohu-rangi was famous for descending to the human realm and taking a lover: a human called Uenuku. He was entranced by her, but she made it utterly clear that she could stay with him only during the hours of darkness. It was imperative that she depart before dawn. She warned him that should he ever reveal her presence and identity to any other human, she would leave him, never to return. Soon after being given this warning, Uenuku was awoken just before dawn by a female voice. As he lay there in the darkness, now fully awake, he heard it again. It seemed to be coming from the peak of the ceiling space above him. The voice called urgently, 'Hine-pūkohu-rangi E! Kua tata ki te awatea' (Hine-pūkohu-rangi! Daylight is almost upon us.). Uenuku had never heard this voice before and was unnerved by it. Wondering if it might be some evil presence, he gently nudged Hine-pūkohu-rangi awake and said, 'Can you hear a voice calling out?' They both listened and there it was again. 'Āe, that's my sister, Hinewai.' She jumped up, dressed herself quickly and departed into the early dawn mist.

Uenuku was hearing a voice calling from the ceiling space, with no apparent person there to explain it. What does this tell us about how my tīpuna (ancestors) viewed disembodied voices? This pūrākau shows that even if you have no clue about the origin of such an experience, there may well be a coherent explanation. And the answer could lie in the realm of wairua. In this case, some say Hinewai is the goddess of light misty rain; others that she is a tūrehu – a particular kind of spirit being. Either way, although invisible to most of humanity, she is considered real. Furthermore, voices can be experienced when you have a kaitiaki or spiritual guardian watching over you – in this case, a caring sister. They can certainly indicate a protective presence. In addition, if you're not sure, asking others for assistance – especially those with spiritual awareness and expertise – can help you make sense of a puzzling experience. For Uenuku, hearing this voice could have been disturbing but Hine-pūkohu-rangi was able to enlighten him and he was no longer troubled by it. The message was hard for Uenuku to decipher because it was not intended for him. For Hine-pūkohu-rangi the message was immediately clear due to her connection with the speaker.

There is more to this story. For some time Uenuku complied with Hine-pūkohu-rangi's insistence that he tell no one about her. However, his pride began to stir, and he longed to tell his friends and whānau (family) about her. Eventually he could no longer contain this yearning and spilled the beans. They refused to believe him at first but urged him to prove his boast. He was persuaded to cover up all the openings in the whare (house) so that she might be tricked into sleeping longer and they could see her for themselves in the morning light (Best, 1972). Upon being revealed, Hine-pūkohu-rangi sang a beautiful waiata (song) lamenting the deception of Uenuku and announcing that she was leaving for good. Uenuku spent the rest of his life grieving his loss and searching for her. The rainbow, so closely associated with mist and rain, is said to be the sign that they were reunited after he left his mortal body.

This cautionary tale counsels about the hazards of getting caught up in what your ego wants for you. Uenuku, in his folly, lost that which was most precious to him. My kuia used to say, 'Me whakaiti koe i a koe.' This means you must always be the least. She taught that humility can protect us in all aspects of life but particularly in the realm of wairua.

Rata and Voice Hearing

Another of our tīpuna from Hawaiki, by the name of Rata, had his own voice-hearing experience that is instructive for related reasons. In order to undertake a long voyage, Rata was given the task of building an ocean-going waka, or vessel. He identified a towering tōtara in the great forest of Tāne, and over the course of a day, felled it with his adze (axe-like tool). When he returned the following morning to begin work on the waka, to his astonishment the tree was upright and totally intact (Ihimaera, 2020). There was no sign that he had even been there the previous day. Nevertheless, he was sure it was the best tree for his purpose and spent the rest of the day cutting it down again. Exhausted, he headed back to his village. Come the next dawn, Rata was onsite at first light. He was shocked to see the tree back to its original vertical and pristine state. However, now he was feeling hōhā (irritated). Ignoring his aching body, he summoned his determination and resumed chopping. By dusk the tree had fallen once more.

This time he resolved to find out who or what was thwarting him. Rata hid nearby and waited. Some hours passed, and he was struggling to stay awake in the dim light. Then he heard voices, singing with an ethereal quality he had never known before. Now they began instructing the tree to repair itself. Immediately the forest was alive with rustling as the tree somehow reassembled itself; then the voices directed it to resume its upright position, and with a great creaking and cracking it did so. Rata was perplexed but also angry. He stepped out of his hiding place. At that moment he found himself face to face with a multitude of forest guardians known as tūrehu. Rata couldn't help himself – he raged at them for foiling all his hard work. The tūrehu listened calmly, and when he had finished his ranting, there was a pause. After some moments, one of them spoke. 'We are the kaitiaki of Te Waonui a Tāne – Tāne's great forest – and you have not sought permission or carried out appropriate karakia (prayers) to be taking one of Tāne's children like this. Where is your respect?'

That stopped Rata in his tracks. Despite his temper, he immediately realised they were right. Feeling quite deflated, he trudged back to his village to consult his elders about what to do next.

When we relate this pūrākau to our kōrero about voice-hearing, what does it teach us about how these experiences were viewed by our tīpuna? To me, the singing Rata hears first reveals the connection these tūrehu have with the realm of wairua, their aroha (love) for the tree and every aspect of their environment. The voice he hears next, directing the tree to rise up, shows us that the tūrehu are in relationship to the tree. Not only that: it seems that they have a connection with every wood chip and particle of it. Every piece is responding to their instruction, presumably under the overall influence of Tāne. This is a very intimate and holistic bond they have with that tree. As a result of that relationship, they have that influence. The final voice Rata hears is the voice of the tūrehu who speaks directly to him. The message from that utterance has profound meaning: not only for Rata, but for all of us.

I like this story. It tells us we will encounter obstacles in our path if we don't take care of wairua. It teaches us about showing respect for the environment and the sacred nature of the tree. It provides a lesson on the importance of using karakia to honour our relationship with Tāne Mahuta (atua of forests).

When Rata first hears the voices singing, he might have wondered if his mind was playing tricks on him. Seeing the wood chips flying back together would have seemed unbelievable. But I doubt he would have thought it was a psychotic experience. He would have known that there was a spiritual realm. He would have heard about tūrehu and their role of protecting the forest. Despite his anger, he would have been curious, even though the experience defied all his logic.

And look at the approach that these tūrehu take to Rata's misdemeanour. They didn't shout back at him or takahi (tread) on his mana (spiritual authority). They explained calmly. Their form of protest was a non-violent one. They were trying to teach him something. I would say that Rata's angry response suggests that he was quite caught up in what his ego was wanting – to get on with building the waka – and he needed to let go of that in order to learn the lesson Tāne and the tūrehu were trying to teach him.

Mātaatua and Seeing a Vision

My kuia had many stories of our ancestors, including adventures across the vast stretches of Te Moana-nui-a-Kiwa (the Pacific Ocean). Our waka on my Tūhoe side was Mātaatua. One narrative that explains its name took place on an early voyage to Aotearoa. The waka got caught in a storm and entered a dangerous whirlpool known as Te Korokoro-o-te-parata (Ihimaera, 2020). Toroa, the captain of the waka, chanted an ancient karakia and somehow the waka was spat out of the whirlpool unharmed. In his gratitude, Toroa gave thanks to the atua and experienced a sudden vision of an ancient mata or face in front of him. He was convinced this was the appearance of the atua that had saved them. He later renamed the vessel in honour of this event, with Mātaatua referring to the face of the atua.

This story demonstrates a common meaning that my kuia would put to experiences such as visions. From her point of view, a vision could represent a true perception of a communication from atua or ancestors who may reveal themselves to strengthen their relationship with the living at a time of crisis. This is a further example of a kaitiaki offering protection. Toroa's vision was an experience that would have been private to him. We can't verify what he experienced, just as we can't know for sure about anyone else's internal experience. Maybe he made it up or the story developed some time after as the events moved into the realm of legend. Perhaps he did see the face, but it was a visual hallucination caused by the stress he was under at the time. Naturally others may be sceptical about such experiences. My view is he most likely had a true perception of his atua or tīpuna appearing to him. This kind of experience is commonly accepted in my culture. I have seen enough visions of my own over the years that I have no trouble accepting this interpretation. You can turn to Chapter 6 for a further example of this kind of vision in Tohu's story.

Visions of Toiroa Ikariki

It's easy to speculate about events from centuries ago. However, is there any historical evidence that our tīpuna have had visions that helped them know things they couldn't have known otherwise? Toiroa Ikariki is an example of an ancestor for whom we have such evidence.

According to East Coast traditions, as a young man in the mid-1760s, Toiroa began having visions so compelling that he set out to visit local kāinga (villages), alerting communities to what he had seen. Toiroa lived in Nukutaurua in Māhia Peninsula, south of Tūranganui-a-Kiwa (the area around Gisborne). Certain of his ancestors were renowned as matakite (seers of future events), giving credibility to his surprising kōrero.

Toiroa warned people about the arrival of strangers whose red-and-white appearance he likened to 'titipa', a striped earthworm (Binney, 1995). He called them 'Pakerewha', which referred to the sickness which their arrival would herald. He described their God, whose son was murdered, foretelling the arrival of Christian missionaries. He indicated that this God was good but there were dark times ahead (NiaNia et al., 2017a).

Toiroa went on to demonstrate what he had seen with pictures in the sand of creatures, objects and garments no locals had ever seen. He drew horses and ships with billowing sails. He fashioned trousers from a cloak and put them on, calling them pūkoro. In those days, men and women wore maro, a garment resembling a short kilt, and piupiu, a longer garment made of flax, for ceremonial occasions; however, covering the legs with material was unheard of. According to Judith Binney (1995), Toiroa wove himself a hat out of flax and showed how it would be worn, calling it 'taupopoki'. He crafted a timber ship with a tiller and ignited flames inside a small black shell in the centre. He named this 'ngatoroirangi' (the fires of heaven). To me, this sure sounds like he was anticipating the coming of steamship technology. Toiroa very deliberately made his way north, speaking to communities about what he had seen, until finally he arrived in Tūranga-nui-a-Kiwa. In 1769, the *Endeavour* made landfall at this exact location and the first Europeans set foot on Aotearoa.

How did Toiroa know all these things? The only explanation that makes sense to me is that he had seen them in wairua. As a matakite, he may have seen them in dreams, or he may have had visions while awake. However, my ancestors didn't make much distinction between these different types of visions. Both were considered important means to receive communication from ancestors and atua.

Other Indigenous cultures have similar understandings and traditions. Around early 1519, in the lead-up to the Spanish invasion of what is now Mexico, there were reports of many local Indigenous people dreaming about the arrival of heavily armed, pale-skinned outsiders. Native American writers also describe visions and dreams as commonly accepted sources of communication from the spirit world (Morse & García, 2021; Mohatt & Eagle Elk, 2000).

Returning to my kuia, I never heard her talk about these visions of Toiroa. However, she was very interested in a prophecy he made about his mokopuna (grandchild), Te Kooti Arikirangi Te Turuki. Toiroa foresaw the life of a child born to one of two cousins in his whānau, who would lead the people in dark times. That child was Te Kooti.

Te Kooti

My kuia told us many stories about Te Kooti. As a young man he learnt to read and write Māori and English at a Wesleyan school, studied the Old Testament and even considered becoming an Anglican priest. He later gained experience as a seaman and as a merchant. A canny businessman, not averse to trickery if it served his purpose, Te Kooti developed enemies amongst local Pākehā (New Zealand European) businessmen. By the mid-1860s he fought as a soldier in East Coast battles between the government and a Māori movement known as the Hauhau rebellion. This was considered a holy war by the rebels, who were fighting against unjust confiscation of land (Walker, 2004). Although Te Kooti fought on the government side, in November 1865, in the midst of this conflict, he was arrested, accused of spying and imprisoned without trial. In June 1866, amongst a shipload of Hauhau prisoners including men, women and children, he was exiled to Wharekauri, the remote Chatham Islands (Binney, 1995). In all, 272 people were imprisoned there.

Māori Land Alienation

In order to understand the situation that Te Kooti was facing, we need to consider a bigger picture. According to Judith Binney (1995), Te Kooti would have been a child of eight years when, in 1840, rangatira (leaders) from many iwi signed the Māori version of Te Tiriti o Waitangi (The Treaty of Waitangi). Māori were already trading with settlers locally and offshore. In many cases, our business interests were thriving in the 1840s (Walker, 2004). However, while Te Tiriti guaranteed those iwi tino rangatiratanga (unqualified authority) over their whenua (land), kaimoana (fisheries), and other resources and taonga (ancestral and cultural treasures), it was soon apparent that the settlers had no intention of honouring those promises. In less than a decade, corrupt negotiators had duped South Island iwi into selling 8 million hectares of land for only £2,000, a transaction known as the Kemp Purchase (Mikaere, 1988). We know Te Kooti had strong views about Māori land alienation as he was involved in protests about these matters in the early 1850s (Binney, 1995).

By the 1860s, it was obvious the government was determined to steal Māori land by deception or force. A blatant example of this was the military invasion of the Waikato by the government in 1863 (Walker, 2004). In this context, the imprisonment of Te Kooti without trial, on a trumped-up charge, is clearly part of a bigger picture of colonial oppression. I sometimes say that the quickest way to kill Māori is to separate us from our whenua. And the process with which it was done showed no respect. For me, this was about takahi of mana. Te Kooti was considered a troublemaker and a threat, so the colonial authorities used their power to remove him.

Rēkohu

For nine years I worked on Rēkohu, which is the Moriori name for Wharekauri, otherwise known as the Chatham Islands, a small group of islands situated 800 kilometres east of the South Island of Aotearoa. Rēkohu refers to the shifting mists prevalent there. I would fly in monthly for several days and see people for mahi wairua (spiritual healing) consultations. Rēkohu is a very spiritual place. It has a flat, windswept landscape with exposed trees that lean towards the horizontal. For some people it might seem desolate, but I saw a rugged beauty there.

I soon learnt about the history of the Moriori iwi, the tāngata whenua, the Indigenous people of Rēkohu. They suffered many atrocities at the hands of another iwi in the 1830s and were almost wiped out. This had a severe impact on the survival of their language, culture and traditions (King, 1989).

I recall my kuia telling stories about Te Kooti's imprisonment there. He arrived with other detainees in the middle of the winter of 1866. Southerly winds direct from the Antarctic would have been bitterly cold. They had inadequate clothing, hardly any food and little shelter. Over the following weeks they were forced to build their own dwellings using ponga (tree fern) and other local timber. By December that year Te Kooti was in very poor health (Binney, 1995). He had a fluctuating fever and had lost a considerable amount of weight. At times he was coughing up blood, which Allister tells me could indicate he had a serious illness such as tuberculosis. By early the following year his condition had deteriorated further. It was reported that 'he was so ill he was taken to a separate whare to die' and a casket was prepared for him (Binney, 1995). By this time, I imagine many of his fellow detainees might have been losing hope they would ever see their whānau and whenua again.

Uncommon Perceptual Experiences

Te Kooti had the first of a series of visions and voice-hearing experiences on 21 February 1867. During a particularly bad episode of fever, he later recalled that 'te wairua o te Atua' or the spirit of God raised him up and spoke to him (Binney, 1995). However, in his diary he wrote that his feverish state meant he was unable to remember the details of what this reo or voice said.

What did Te Kooti experience here? Was his imagination running away with him in his confused, feverish state? Was he having a psychotic episode? Did he make this up later to convince his followers that he had a special relationship with God? Or was he having a spiritual experience? I find his description interesting. I don't think he would bother to say he couldn't recall what the voice said if he made it up to impress his followers. When I have seen something in the wairua during a healing session with a person, I am always very careful to sit with that until I am sure about how to make sense of what I have seen. If I'm not sure, I won't say anything. To me, this detail suggests Te Kooti is being careful about the accuracy of his description. And something about this experience is very compelling for him. Despite his severe illness, he resolves to keep a careful diary from that time forth.

Diary

Given that he has grown up in te ao Māori, where knowledge was passed down orally, why does Te Kooti decide to keep a diary? In the Ngāti Maru iwi he was born into, written language may have been unknown in his early years. However, by his young adulthood he was a fluent reader and writer of te reo and English. He must have decided that written language could be an effective way to document his experience accurately and would allow him to communicate with others even at a distance, over time and space.

My tipuna Tūtakangahau was a paramount chief of Tamakaimoana, a hapū (subtribe) of Ngāi Tūhoe. Born around 1830, he lived deep in Te Urewera near our sacred mountain, Maungapōhatu. There were no roads, and very few Europeans would have entered that area before 1840. However, around that time an informal mission school was set up in Tūtakangahau's village by a Catholic priest. There Tūtakangahau and a number of his whānau learnt to read and write te reo (Best, 1972). At first, my tipuna was not convinced that written language was useful. He later explained that he and his whānau tested it many times by writing a message and sending it to a distant place to be read by 'unseen persons'. In later life, it is clear Tūtakangahau had realised there was value in the ability to write. He lobbied government officials by corresponding with them directly. He expressed his views in Māori language newspapers. Years later, in 1895, he approached Elsdon Best, a self-taught Pākehā anthropologist, to record Ngāi Tūhoe – the whakapapa (genealogy), karakia, histories and other traditions of the Tūhoe nation – in written form, so it would be available for future generations (Holman, 2010). Tūtakangahau gave refuge to Te Kooti when the militia was pursuing him. He would have known that Te Kooti was a matakite and would have heard about his visions and voice-hearing experiences. I am confident that my tipuna held Te Kooti in high regard. Matakite experiences would have been part of my ancestor's world view.

Voice

The next recorded experience of Te Kooti occurred one month after the first incident. On 21 March 1867, his diary entry recounts that he became unconscious again. Upon regaining awareness, he heard exactly the same voice speaking to him as he had heard before. The historical records describe how his friends were 'weeping over him' (Binney, 1995). I assume they thought he was close to death. When he asked them who had spoken, they said they didn't hear anything. Te Kooti then concluded it was God speaking to him. Without being there myself, it's impossible for me to say if it really was God speaking to him. However, I am satisfied that people do have those encounters. Such experiences may take many forms. To me, Te Kaihanga, The Creator, is not limited to one people, or one time, or one place. In my view, it is possible that Te Kooti really did hear the voice of God.

Vision

On 21 April of the same year, Te Kooti wrote that he had lost consciousness once more and on waking could hear the same voice he had heard on those two previous occasions. The reo told him 'kaua e wehi' (don't be overawed); that God had heard his plea and would teach him words spoken to 'koutou tipuna' (all your ancestors) (Binney, 1995). Then the voice appeared to him as a dramatic vision. According to Te Kooti's account, written in te reo, the figure he saw appeared to be walking on a white cloud, their kākahu (clothing) as white as snow, their māhunga (head) surrounded by stars with the sun as their crown. He described the figure's tokotoko (staff) as emanating a power beyond anything he had ever witnessed, with the rays of the sun like darts fanning out on each side. It is clear that Te Kooti believed he was kanohi ki te kanohi, or face to face with Te Atua, or God. In his kōrero he was trying to find language to express the awesomeness of this encounter.

Te Kooti is not just a bit roughed up; he has been imprisoned in a cold, desolate place and is severely ill. You could say he is being crushed by circumstances. At this moment he has an experience that seems to change his whole outlook. I would speculate that at this low point in Te Kooti's life, due to his vulnerability, there is an opening. He was most likely a man with a strong sense of himself and a robust ego. There is a saying, 'Tēnei te pō, nau mai te ao.' To me, this means, 'At our darkest moments, we may find the light we need.' Perhaps it took this set of circumstances, these obstacles, for an aperture to open up – he kūaha (a moment of openness) – at which time Te Kooti is emotionally and spiritually available to receive an experience that connects him with his Source. He hears a voice and sees a vision of a figure filled with light and begins to feel an intense sense of connection with Te Kaihanga.

In reflecting on Te Kooti's situation, what can we learn from the fruits of his experiences? After this time, his writing indicates he has a new purpose: he has faith in Te Atua, which he interprets as the God of Abraham and the prophets of the Old Testament. Having previously been close to death, his health begins to steadily improve. He takes on a new role in leading others in spiritual practices. He has hope that life can be different despite the devastating effects of the colonial authority's oppression of his people. He plans and leads an escape from Rēkohu onboard a ship called the *Rifleman* and returns to his ancestral lands. Here, he and his followers are pursued by colonial militia. This pursuit continues for some years, and he is engaged in resistance against the Crown. Many people, Māori and Pākehā, lost their lives during that time. However, Te Kooti never lost sight of his faith and spiritual purpose, and his teachings became the foundation for Te Hāhi Ringatū – the Ringatū faith.

Te Hāhi Ringatū

In the Wairoa district, south of Gisborne, up the Ruakituri valley, there is a very old marae (Māori meeting house) called Paraeroa which was set aside for Te Hāhi Ringatū. The word 'hā' is the breath and the word 'hi' means to raise. So 'hāhi' means to raise to life. Ringatū refers to the upraised hand which was a symbol of this faith. This is about acknowledgement or acceptance of submission to the divine Source. My kuia and my koroua (male elder) were both Ringatū followers. I was baptised Ringatū when I was very young. On 'tekau mā rua', the 12th of every month, our whānau would travel in my Dad's dark green Wolseley sedan: my kuia, my koroua and three of us kids, with the others all at boarding school. We would leave home in the afternoon and arrive at the marae. Formalities would commence with a whakatau (welcome), then we would have kai (food). After this the church event would start and continue late into the evening. Ringatū ceremonies involve long, solemn recitation of karakia and chanting of waiata, often over many hours. There may have been 40 or 50 people or more. There would have been several Ringatū ministers. This is the church Te Kooti started, and it all started with those voices and visions he experienced. The Ringatū religion is still strong today and offers spiritual sustenance to a lot of people.

As a young child I found the formal proceedings monotonous, but the stories that my kuia told about Te Kooti's life captured my imagination. I was enraptured as she recounted tales of Te Kooti's exploits as a rebel, resisting the colonial authorities and evading the pursuing militia. He was one of my heroes.

Understanding Te Kooti's Experiences

My formal education finished when I left school at the age of 13. I am no academic or psychiatrist. There are several ways to interpret what Te Kooti heard and saw. It's possible he was hallucinating due to a delirious state. But when I consider the fruits of his experience, and my own experiences of Te Kaihanga, I consider it more likely that he was having spiritual experiences. In te ao Māori, many people would accept that visions can come from a spiritual source, which could include tīpuna, other entities or even a divine connection.

Rua Kēnana

In the last years of his life, Te Kooti made a prediction that a new leader would come from the land of the Mātaatua waka (Binney, 1990). This area includes Te Urewera, where Rua Kēnana was born. He lived initially at Maungapōhatu but then moved to be with his father's whānau in Hawke's Bay. He later returned to the area of his birth, working as a shearer and labourer.

It's important to remember the extreme circumstances our Tūhoe people were facing at the turn of the century. Two hundred thousand hectares of Tūhoe land were confiscated by the government in the late 1860s (Waitangi

Tribunal, 2009). During the pursuit of Te Kooti by the colonial militia, homes and crops were destroyed and people and livestock killed. Introduced diseases contributed to further deaths and demoralisation of our communities. Further land dispossession as a result of the unjust Native Land Court led to worsening poverty. In the five years leading up to 1901, the Tūhoe population dropped from 1,400 to 1,000 (Binney et al., 1979).

By 1905, Rua was living with his wife, Pinepine, in a whare made from ponga very near Maungapōhatu. He later described how he was interrupted while making bread by a voice calling him (Binney et al., 1979). He turned around and asked his wife if she had called him, but she said she hadn't. This question suggests to me that Rua was hearing a voice emanating from outside of his personal space. This distinction is not one that I focus on much because I hear voices that come from both inside and outside of me. For example, the voice I heard on the road to Mahia in Chapter 1 sounded like it came from the inside of the car I was in, but outside of myself. Other times, it may be hard to tell the difference. But in this instance, the fact that Rua asked Pinepine that question makes it clear he was hearing an external voice. The voice then called him again. I expect by now he was curious. When the voice called him a third time, he went outside to investigate. He must have thought the voice came from outside the house. As soon as he got out there, he saw a figure that he deduced was an angelic being. This makes me wonder how he knew that. Without asking him, it's hard to tell. His conclusion suggests to me a Christian influence. But it also makes me think this figure must have identified itself to him in some way. However, I would be interested to know what made Rua decide the being he saw was angelic.

This was his first vision. The angel told him to ascend the sacred mountain Maungapōhatu. He and Pinepine set off and began their walk up the steep track. After some time, their path became shrouded in mist and increasingly difficult to follow. The tradition tells that three times they became exhausted from their climbing and stopped to rest, wondering if they were lost. Each time a woman with long black hair appeared to them and showed them the way. From this account, it seems both Rua and Pinepine were having the same vision. Rua came to know that she was Whaitiri, a well-known Tūhoe ancestor. When they finally reached the top, she showed herself again. This time, alongside Whaitiri, Rua saw a figure he identified as Jesus Christ.

I am confident that Rua was matekite (spiritually aware). As such, he would most likely have had visions of deceased ancestors from time to time. Being matekite myself, I know it can happen. Seeing people who have passed on can be just as vivid for me as seeing a living person. Sometimes I find it hard to tell the difference. If it was one of my own ancestors, I would usually know. Even if I am seeing someone else's ancestor, sometimes I might see them and their name may just come to me as happened in Tohu's story in Chapter 6. It makes sense to me that if Rua was seeing his ancestor, he could have recognised who she was. As regards to him seeing Jesus Christ, I have known a number of people who have been sure that they have seen Christ. Such an experience could come from Te Kaihanga and could be part of matekite, as far as I'm concerned.

What can we say about the fruits of these experiences? Again, let us consider the saying 'Mā te hua ka kitea': by the fruits we can see more clearly. Following these experiences, Rua travelled around Te Urewera, explaining what he had seen. As a result, he was accepted by many Tūhoe as being the leader that Te Kooti had foretold. At a desolate time, Rua inspired hope in our people. In 1907 he established a settlement on Maungapōhatu and persuaded as many as 600 followers to join him there. Rua was the mokopuna of Tūtakangahau, and my tipuna joined him at Maungapōhatu in the last years of his life. It was a spiritual community. Rua was aiming for a peaceful and self-sufficient existence, separated off from Pākehā interference (Walker, 2004). The community cleared land for farming and orchards, brought in livestock and established a clean water supply and careful hygiene standards. It settled its own disputes. It built a school to educate its children. However, the government was disturbed by Rua's rejection of its authority, his claim to be a new Messiah and his prediction that Pākehā would be expelled out of Aotearoa. His activities as a Māori healer also attracted hostile responses from the government and contributed to calls to ban such practices.

If we return to the theme of this book, what are we to make of the visions and voices that Rua experienced? Whether or not you agree with everything that Rua said or did, there is nothing in the historical accounts, aside from his visions and voice-hearing experiences, to suggest he was suffering from a psychotic illness. He was very well organised in the way he led the people. If he had been suffering from a significant psychiatric problem, I don't expect Tūhoe would have taken his claims seriously. If his spiritual authority was stronger as a result of what he said about his visions and voices, then that supports what I am saying; in my culture, these kinds of experiences have been known as part of wairua going way back.

Tohunga Suppression Act

In 1907, the government passed legislation to ban the activities of tohunga (Māori healers). The Tohunga Suppression Act outlawed

> every person who gathers Maoris [*sic*] around him by practicing on their superstition or credulity, or who misleads or attempts to mislead any Maori by professing or pretending to possess supernatural powers in the treatment or cure of any disease, or in the foretelling of future events.
>
> (Durie, 1998: p. 44)

This law had far-reaching negative consequences for Māori healing. People feared that they would be imprisoned or their land would be confiscated if it became known they were practicing tohungatanga (Māori expertise). Whare wānanga or schools of Māori healing were closed or driven underground, and mātauranga Māori was discredited and lost. Even after the repeal of this unjust legislation in the mid-1960s, many of our people had lost their connection to this realm of Māori healing knowledge.

The Assault on Maungapōhatu

Meanwhile, Pākehā authorities were looking for other reasons to arrest Rua. He had openly opposed a dog tax that he said was unfairly targeting Māori communities (Walker, 2004). He also objected to legislation making it illegal for Māori – but not for Pākehā – to buy alcohol for consumption at home. Even though Rua wasn't encouraging Māori to drink alcohol, the result of this law was that Pākehā were making a lot of money from Māori communities by supplying illicit grog (alcohol) (Walker, 2004). At the onset of World War I, Rua was vocal in discouraging Tūhoe men from volunteering for the armed services. This was due to his commitment to peace and his view that this foreign war was not relevant to Māori. The government accused him of inciting rebellion against the Crown. However, because that wasn't illegal, they decided to arrest him on a historic charge of sly-grogging (selling alcohol without a licence). On 2 April 1916, 60 heavily armed police on foot and horseback marched up to the settlement at Maungapōhatu to apprehend Rua. Although he had instructed his followers to greet the police peacefully, and kai had been prepared to welcome them, the police confronted him with firearms. In the resulting scuffle, shots were fired, and two young Māori men from the settlement were murdered (Binney et al., 1979). Rua himself was assaulted. My kuia was there that day. I never heard her talk about this incident when I was young. It was many years later when I once heard her speak of it. Her whānau were visiting Maungapōhatu from Rūātoki the day the police arrived. When the men were shot, she was hiding under a whare with some of the other children. She was terrified that she would be dragged out from under the house and killed. I could tell that she had been carrying that mamae (hurt) all those years. I sometimes wonder if the trauma of events like that could have contributed to some of her health problems.

Down-to-Earth Wairua Experiences

Almost all of the written descriptions of Māori voice-hearing and visions pertain to our Māori prophets. Most of them focus on experiences that they or others considered important in establishing their spiritual authority.

There are very few accounts of everyday matekite and matakite experiences. What gets written about are often experiences of angelic beings or communication from Te Kaihanga. Many of these accounts use language that seems to line up with the Bible. I think this gives a distorted picture. In my life, wairua experiences are normal and common. My kuia also talked about everyday wairua as normal. It puzzles me that there are so few down-to-earth stories documented about seeing tīpuna, or about someone who has passed away coming back to say goodbye. There are very few narratives of people having a premonition, or sensing sickness in another person, when it was not apparent to others.

One reason I believe they weren't written down is that in te ao Māori, these experiences have been considered normal and ordinary. Maybe Māori writers didn't think it was worth documenting them because everyone knew those things could happen. On the other hand, it's also likely they weren't recorded because Māori believed these experiences would be frowned on by Christianity or other Pākehā authorities. I expect most Pākehā authors wouldn't write them down because these stories wouldn't line up with their worldview. At the same time, many Pākehā I have met have told me about their own wairua experiences. I wonder if they would be reluctant to write about these experiences because of the mainstream viewpoint that wairua experiences are not considered scientific and are therefore assumed to be not valid.

One exception in the literature was a description by a woman from Rua's settlement at Maungapōhatu. She described seeing 'kēhua' (ghosts) dancing and passing through the windows of a whare after the two men were killed there (Binney et al., 1979).

Another story relates to a visionary and prophet from Te Waipounamu (the South Island) called Hipa Te Maiharoa (Mikaere, 1988). He was affiliated with Kāi Tahu, Kāti Māmoe and Waitaha iwi. In 1877 he led a heke or migration of many of his followers more than 100 miles inland to Ōmarama, in the southern Canterbury region, where they occupied ancestral land in protest against the injustice of the Kemp Purchase. In August 1879, he ascended Mauka Atua, the highest point on the Ben Ohau range, a sacred mountain to his people. There he experienced a vision from which he concluded that a new home for his people would be Korotuaheka, at the mouth of the Waitaki River (Mikaere, 1988). I am not aware of further documentation of the details of that vision. However, after the move to Korotuaheka, there was an incident in which he experienced a vision of a more ordinary sort.

Te Paro, a member of Hipa Te Maiharoa's community, reported that one day Te Maiharoa stormed out of his whare to confront some of his followers who were returning to the village (Mikaere, 1988). He accused these men of stealing and killing some pigs from a nearby settler. As evidence he insisted that he could see Pākehā pigs following them, which no one else could see. He then contacted the police. The offenders were later arrested when it was confirmed that the pigs had indeed been taken and killed. Clearly Te Maiharoa had seen something in the wairua that revealed to him what they had done. And his experience was validated by the findings of the police in their investigation.

Hohepa Kereopa, a tohunga from Waimana in Te Urewera and one of Rua's relatives, was also a Tūhoe relation of mine. He explained that when he heard voices that other people couldn't hear he could always identify a body to go with it. He gave the following example:

> One time, I heard someone behind me, and I saw an old lady wearing a cardigan over her shoulders, and she said that everything was all right. And I thought to myself, 'Now, who wears a cardigan like that?' And then I remembered. It was one of my aunties. And that afternoon, I got the phone call. She had passed away.
>
> (Moon, 2003: pp.109–110)

I believe Kereopa's description is an excellent example of a common Māori experience around the time of someone's death. I myself have had many experiences like that.

Mere Rikiriki and Other Wāhine Prophets

I know of very few written descriptions of voice-hearing and visions from wāhine (women). Yet I would say that women are just as spiritual as men, perhaps more so.

Judith Binney (1990) wrote about three women prophets from the far north who were active in the Hokianga in the 1880s. They were Maria and Remana Pangari and Ani Kaaro. However, I am not aware of any detailed accounts of their experiences.

At the same time that Rua was leading his community at Maungapōhatu, a female prophet from a different whakapapa line was becoming known in Taranaki. An earlier rangatira and prophet, Te Kere Ngātai-e-rua, had erected a wooden cross on the wharenui (ancestral meeting house) at Te Takinga by the Rangitīkei River, in Te Ika-a-Māui (the North Island). During a period of illness at the end of his life, Te Kere announced that whoever the cross fell on would inherit his healing and prophetic mantle. It fell on Mere Rikiriki (Young, 1998). She became sought-after as a healer and used rongoā (herbal medicines) as part of her treatment. However, she avoided accusations of tohungatanga in those early years after the Tohunga Suppression Act by carrying out her mahi (work) in the name of the holy spirit. She was said to have a room filled with crutches no longer required by those she had healed. She always said, 'Pray to God, not to me, for I am only an instrument' (Newman, 2009: p22). She was known as the 'prophetess of peace', emphasised the unity of Māori under one God and advocated for the honouring of Te Tiriti o Waitangi.

I have no doubt that Mere Rikiriki was a very spiritual person. I expect that she may have had many wairua experiences. However, I am not aware of any written documentation of these. In 1912, she foretold the coming of a tāne (man) in her whānau whom the 'wairua' or spirit of prophecy would enter (Binney, 1990).

Tahupōtiki Wiremu Rātana

Tahupōtiki Wiremu Rātana was in his mid-40s in 1918 when he first began having strange and unusual experiences. Affiliated with Ngāti Apa iwi, he had grown up on whānau land just south of the Whanganui River, in the central part of Te Ika-a-Māui. As a young man Rātana worked as a ploughman, a wheat-stacker and a fencer (Newman, 2009). He often attended his Aunty Mere's church and would have known of her healing mahi. Although he was encouraged to become a minister as a young adult, instead he continued his life as a farmer with his wife, Te Urumanao, and children. He had a keen interest in horse racing, acted as a bookmaker and enjoyed drinking with friends at the local bar.

Rātana's life changed following a series of events in 1918. The first was a whānau fishing expedition to the mouth of a local river. Rātana and the whānau were astonished when two whales washed up on the beach directly in front of them. Twelve days later, his three-year-old son, Omeka, was injured and developed a knee infection. The boy's condition fluctuated but after a number of months, he became severely ill. On 8 November that year, Rātana was standing on his veranda, considering whether his son should be admitted to hospital. As he looked out towards the moana (ocean), he noticed a distinctive cloud in the distance. It was dark on the edges but pure white in the centre and flame-like at the rear. He watched intently as it moved steadily towards him. By the time it was directly overhead, the cloud split open, and Rātana suddenly felt 'overwhelmed by its presence' (Newman, 2009; p33). At that moment he had his first vision. He could see many trails, paths and highways from all corners of the world leading to his whare. Over the next hours, his whānau became increasingly concerned by his behaviour. In one instance he leapt onto a table in the kitchen and declared, 'Peace be upon you; for I am the Holy Spirit who is speaking to you' (Newman, 2009: p33). He told them to prepare themselves. If a psychiatrist had seen this, it wouldn't surprise me if they might have interpreted his behaviour as psychotic at that moment. But it is interesting to reflect on what happened next: what the fruits of these experiences were as time went on.

Within three days of these experiences, World War 1 ended in Europe. Rātana told his whānau that a voice had told him they should leave their homes, as disaster was about to strike. Meanwhile, the influenza epidemic of 1918 had reached Aotearoa. Those of his family who stayed at home all died of influenza, but his mother and nephew – who had followed his advice – were unaffected. If they had dismissed his kōrero as psychotic, they would likely have perished. Over the following weeks, Rātana frequently heard the same voice, which identified itself as Ihoa (God). The voice told him that he would become 'Te Māngai', the mouthpiece of Ihoa, and that his followers would become known as 'Ngā Mōrehu' (the survivors).

During this time, Omeka became more unwell and had an operation to try to address his knee infection. After this his condition worsened further, and Rātana and Te Urumanao decided to bring him home. They spent three days fasting, praying and caring for him. Rātana again heard the same voice telling him his son would be cured. Omeka's leg began to heal, and over time he recovered fully. This incident was considered the first sign of Rātana's healing mahi (Newman, 2009).

My wife, Lesley, is from Te Whānau-a-Apanui. Her great-uncle, Eruera Stirling, described his own experience of visiting Wiremu Rātana in 1919 (Stirling & Salmond, 1980). His mother, Mihi Kōtukutuku, had been diagnosed with terminal breast cancer. She had a large breast lump and had become very unwell. Her doctor gave her a few months to live, at best. Her husband heard that Rātana had been faith healing and decided to take the whānau down to see him. It was a long journey to Whanganui by boat, bus and train. Upon their arrival there were many sick people. They witnessed a young Pākehā woman who had been paralysed from the waist down getting up out of her stretcher and walking after Rātana prayed over her. Eruera Stirling recounted how his mother went up to be blessed by Rātana. He prayed for her and told her that she would be okay. She returned home and sought other rongoā treatment as well. Her breast lump began to shrink and over time seemed to disappear entirely. She went on to live for many years before a recurrence of her breast cancer in the 1950s led to her death in 1956.

Voices, Visions and Healing

I have chosen to retell this story of Mihi Kōtukutuku to illustrate a connection between wairua experiences and Māori healing. In te ao Māori, voices and visions can indicate a potential for healing. Rātana had begun to see and hear things. The content of many of his experiences suggested he had a special connection with Te Kaihanga. There are many accounts that confirm he now had a gift that allowed him to heal others (Newman, 2009).

He helped many people transform their lives: physically as well as spiritually. People who were paralysed or terminally ill got miraculously healed. A lot of people went away with hope.

Rātana was a humble man. It plagued him that people became so focused on him. The idea of Te Māngai, the mouthpiece, is that you are not the source of the message. I believe Rātana was just a human being. The healing came from beyond him. I liken this to a hose with water running through it. Rātana was like that hose, with waiora or healing water flowing through. What was coming through him was healing energy from Wairua: from that divine Source.

Many other Māori healers I have heard of have had the ability to make use of guidance they have received from voices and visions. In my healing mahi I'm guided by particular voices at times, and I have learned to trust that guidance. I believe it is possible that Rātana made use of specific visions and voices to guide his healing work.

Māori Healing versus Western Medicine

The only account I'm aware of describing a direct comparison between Māori healing and Western medicine dates back to the 1870s. It took place near Rotorua, in the North Island of Aotearoa. One dark night, an English soldier visiting that area fell into a hot water spring and sustained severe scalds to both legs up to his hips (Mair, 1923). His host, a local rangatira, advised that Māori healing approaches should be used to address his burns. However, a medical practitioner who examined him insisted that he be treated with the best Western medical methods. Both sides were adamant. Finally, a compromise was reached in which his right leg was to be treated using Māori healing methods and his left leg using the latest Western approaches. His hosts proceeded with a treatment used for many generations in their rohe (area). They collected black mud from the bottom of a local swamp and covered his right leg from hip to toe. After three days it had dried out and started to crack and so he was carried to a nearby healing pool and his right leg was bathed. More black mud was then obtained, and the process was repeated. Meanwhile, lime juice and linseed oil was applied to the skin of his left leg and it was bandaged by his doctor. The patient described the Māori treatment as soothing and much less painful. It was soon clear that his right leg was healing more rapidly. It was completely healed after five weeks. His left leg required several more weeks of the Western treatment.

Despite the clear advantages of this Māori healing approach, there is no indication that the benefits were acknowledged by the Western medical practitioners who witnessed it. This was consistent with prevailing Western attitudes to Māori healing. Any observed benefit was dismissed and there was no interest in investigating it further. It makes me wonder how Māori healing might have progressed if there had been research and development funding available. However, as we know, the opposite took place, and Māori healing was outlawed.

Voices and Visions in Cousins

Patricia Grace is a Māori writer who has whakapapa connections to Ngāti Raukawa, Ngāti Toa Rangatira and Te Ati Awa. Her book *Cousins* offers us another kūaha or entry point into how our culture understands wairua. It tells the story of three kōtiro (girl) cousins, Makareta, Missy and Mata, who grow up under very different circumstances in Aotearoa in the years after World War II.

Later in life, after many years of not seeing each other, Makareta and Mata are reunited. Shortly after this, Makareta becomes unwell and is diagnosed with terminal cancer. She invites Mata to come and live with her in the last months of her life. Mata is surprised at the way Makareta describes her relationship with her deceased grandmother Kui. Makareta explains, 'She's by me. I can't see her, but sometimes she leans on me, sometimes she tickles my arm letting me know she is there. I hear her talking into my mind' (Grace, 1992; p246). It is clear to me from this description that Makareta is spiritually aware of the presence of her grandmother. There is such physical intimacy expressed in those words: a familiar voice heard at the same time as a tactile experience signifying the affection that only her grandmother would have shown her. This very coherent experience confirms for Makareta that her tipuna is really there. To me, this is a typical example of the communication from a loving tipuna. You can read about another example of this in Jake's story in Chapter 8, and Caleb's in Chapter 10.

Not long after this time, Makareta passes away. Mata is alone with her in their whare when it happens, but she soon becomes dimly aware of an old lady in the dark of the room where her cousin is lying. She recognises her from many years before as their grandmother. Then she can see other shadowy figures who look like her and her cousin, 'rustling and shuffling and seating themselves' (Grace, 1992; 247).

After this, the whānau come and take the tūpāpaku (body of the deceased) back north to their home marae, hundreds of miles away. This is Mata's first return since a holiday visit when she was young. Just as they are entering the marae, the kuia begins to karanga for them. Mata describes,

> Something was happening, because suddenly the place became more and more crowded. Suddenly there were people sitting by where the mats had been lain, where at first there had been nobody. There were

> men and women with marked chins and faces who belonged to an older time. They had my own face some of them. Makareta's and mine.
>
> (Grace, 1992; p 254)

Karanga is the ritual calling onto the marae of the manuhiri, or visitors. What follows is a responding call. Traditionally the karanga was always performed by a woman who had given birth. It is said that the cry of a woman giving birth pierces even into the spiritual realm. A woman who had experienced childbirth could therefore be considered for this role. I would say that the karanga can open up a portal to te ao wairua (the spiritual realm).

Even though it's not clear that Mata has been having wairua experiences early in her life, it seems that the death of her cousin and, later, her arrival at her home marae open up a kūaha, a doorway into the spiritual realm. In these moments she is able to see not just one but many of her tīpuna. While those experiences may have been perplexing for Mata at those moments, their origin is to be found in wairua. Even though these examples come from a work of fiction, they are well-recognised scenarios in my culture.

Ā Wairua

The story of the moment of Makareta's death reminds me of a state that my kuia used to call 'ā wairua'. I would translate that expression as meaning 'belonging to or pertaining to wairua'. This is a particular moment when a person is dying, when a kūaha opens up and they start interacting with close whānau members who have previously passed away. In my life, one example occurred when my elder sister, Pare, was dying about 15 years ago. One day, in the last week of her life, I was sitting with her in her room with a few close whānau members. She was lying on her bed. She knew we were there. She was conscious and able to communicate with us. But she was weak and was resting. At that point, I noticed a change in her āhua (appearance). Her face became more animated and she suddenly called out, 'Oh! Hello Aunty!'

Her exclamation took me by surprise. There was a sense of longing in her voice. It sounded like she was greeting a long-lost loved one. Her eyes were open now and she was looking beyond us. I knew she was engaging with someone in the wairua but I couldn't see them myself. However, after some moments, it felt to me like there were others in the room with us. I couldn't actually see them, but it began to feel busy, like there was a crowd gathering in there. I could make out subtle noises in that room that may not have been apparent to others. I could sense sounds like movement, like clothing rubbing past furniture, the creaking of a chair, shoes scuffing on the carpet. I could hear voices speaking in hushed tones but couldn't make out what they were saying. I sensed a feeling of anticipation in that room, and it wasn't coming from those of us who were physically present. It felt to me like the moment on a marae just before the beginning of a pōwhiri (ceremonial welcome). It was as if a welcoming committee had arrived to prepare for my sister's passing.

This phenomenon of 'ā wairua' has been described to me by many others. I have heard scientists attempt to explain behaviour like Pare's away as the final bursts of brain cells firing as the person dies. Perhaps they are suggesting the dying person may be hallucinating. However, my experience told me that in Pare's case, she was being welcomed by our deceased whānau members. They had come to pōwhiri her – to guide her in her transition beyond the veil.

I don't think Pare was afraid to die. She may have been sad to leave her mokopuna behind. She was already aware of wairua and that her tīpuna were with her. She was a staunch Catholic, but she would have been very aware of her tīpuna. Even though I didn't ask Pare what she could see or hear, I'm confident that she was hearing and seeing her tīpuna in wairua.

Wairua experiences around the time of someone's death can take many forms. The word 'kū' is translated in the dictionary as an inarticulate sound. However, this kupu (word) always reminds me of my kuia and the many occasions when she would get into a kū. At these times, she would be asleep in bed late at night and I would be woken by her crying out in her sleep. And this was not a normal cry of distress. Te kū is a keening sound, like the sound women make at a tangihanga (bereavement ritual). It is a heart-wrenching, wailing sound. My kuia believed that people who were about to pass on were visiting to farewell her prior to their death. In some cases, they were trying to take her with them. During those moments there were often cupboard and wardrobe doors opening and closing by themselves in her room, which really freaked me out. It was my job at eight years old to sit with her to help keep her awake and with us. She would try to resist them, but it was as if she was being pulled back into this unconscious state. This would continue for some hours. Finally, often by 6 AM, she would tell us to get up and pack the truck. By the time the phone call came with the news of their death, we were all packed and ready. We would then depart for the tangihanga. As you can see, my kuia educated me about wairua in a number of ways, but the lessons were seldom as exhausting and scary as those middle-of-the-night vigils. This is an example of a kūaha or portal that I suppose was uninvited but, at the same time, part of her gift.

Colonisation, Voices and Visions

There is no one truth about the nature of experiences such as voices or visions. However, as Māori we are very used to having our experiences interpreted for us by outsiders. I expect it is the same for other Indigenous peoples.

In this chapter, we have already seen examples of colonisation of our people in Aotearoa in the stories of Te Kooti, Rua, Te Maiharoa and others. Most people associate colonisation of Indigenous peoples with forced confiscation of ancestral lands by war or legal means, or with the loss of life from killing us or from introduced diseases. But of course there have been many more subtle ways (Royal, 2003). In Aotearoa, the banning of Māori language in schools and other practices of assimilation were designed to shape us as Māori into Pākehā ways of thinking. The Tohunga Suppression Act outlawed our Māori healing practices. When you try to knock my belief systems out of me, that's trying to kill off a culture.

I have explained previously that a koroua (male elder) standing on a marae, holding their rākau (ceremonial staff), has authority to speak. No one will interrupt as long as he has that rākau (NiaNia et al., 2017b). Very often Māori in mental health settings have had that rākau taken away from them. When Māori have been admitted to mental health units, due to their distress, they may be having disturbing experiences in the wairua. I'm not denying that sometimes wairua experiences are difficult to distinguish from psychotic experiences. However, if a Māori rangatahi (youth) in hospital says that they can see their deceased Nanny talking to them, and that is interpreted as a psychotic experience by the clinical team, I would ask, did they have an opportunity for a wairua practitioner to see them? If that is not available to them, then I would ask, how is wairua being attended to? When my Māori world views are not held in mind by mental health professionals, what is the impact on my identity as Māori?

In these ways, I suggest that mental health systems continue to contribute to the silencing of Māori and other Indigenous perspectives. To my way of thinking, this process constitutes a more insidious form of colonisation of our minds as Māori.

Taha wairua (spiritual side) is said to be one of the four quadrants of wellbeing, alongside tinana (physical), hinengaro (psychological), and whānau (relational). In te ao Māori, it is often considered the foundation of everything else (Durie, 1998). Wairua is part of who we are. But frequently this quadrant has been ignored in the training of mental health professionals. The view is that wairua is not scientific. If you can't see it, hold it in your hands, cut it up or pull it to bits, then it doesn't exist. Wairua is like the wind. You can't see the wind, but you can feel it on your cheek. With the sun, you can't see the heat in the air, but you can feel it on your skin.

In our previous book, Allister and I described the story of a young person in distress whose deceased Nanny I could see (NiaNia et al., 2017a). We have also written about a young person called Tangi who was hearing voices screaming at her and was so distressed that she was admitted to an adolescent psychiatry inpatient unit (NiaNia et al., 2017a). I would say that she was experiencing a state of kahupō. She was overwhelmed by those alienating experiences. She wasn't able to see a way out of her predicament. Her psychiatrist made a diagnosis of depression and psychosis. However, in that situation I was also able to perceive the entity that was screaming at her. By working closely with the psychiatry and nursing teams on the unit, it was possible for her treatment to include psychiatric medication and psychological, family and wairua approaches alongside each other. Over time we supported her to take charge of her spiritual and other circumstances, and we placed the rākau firmly back in her hands. Tangi is the artist who provided the artwork for the cover of this book.

Recently I have noticed there are mental health clinicians who are more open to looking at wairua alongside other aspects of their mahi. I have noticed acknowledgement in the mental health training of nurses, social workers, psychologists and psychiatrists that wairua has a significant place. I am aware of psychiatrists and psychologists who are seeing beyond the DSM-5: who are looking into that other quadrant and considering wairua (American Psychiatric Association, 2013). These changes give me hope.

In order to support more clinicians and whānau in understanding the nature of wairua in the context of Māori mental wellbeing, I am keen that more of this kōrero is put on paper. Tūtakangahau recognised the need for our taonga tuku iho – the knowledge handed down to us from our ancestors – to be documented. He wanted it to be available to our mokopuna and others who wish to understand. Just as my tipuna did before me, I want as many people as possible to have access to this kōrero.

3 Ngā Tōpito o te Ao

Wiremu NiaNia, Allister Bush, and David Epston

Wiremu

The title of this chapter, Ngā Tōpito o te Ao, is a phrase that my koroua (male elder) Huatahi often used on our marae when he was referring to people who had come from far places. It means the farthest places of the world. Geographically, the opposite side of the planet from us here in Aotearoa is in Europe. In this chapter we will be looking at stories from a few people on that continent over a time period spanning many generations. Each of them had their own experiences of seeing visions or hearing voices or both.

There is another expression, 'he rerekētanga o te whakaaro', which refers to differing opinions that might pertain to a person's experience. In each story we discuss, there have been very different interpretations of the experiences they described. We are not saying that there is only one point of view. Most European mystics over the centuries have been Christian in their faith and beliefs, and this is reflected in the examples we outline in this chapter. However, we are not saying that Christianity has more validity than any other faith. We are certainly not wanting to tell anyone what to believe spiritually. We all come to this moment with our own life experience and our own worldviews, and everyone is entitled to draw their own conclusions. We all experience the journey differently.

My own perspective is that wairua (spirituality) transcends all space and time. Even though the people we will hear about came from very different cultures to my own, for me the wairua in their stories shines through. Even with accounts from many generations ago, I would say that the wairua that flows through them does not go out of date.

Allister

At the time I completed my medical training, I fully understood the idea that voices and visions could represent a medical, psychiatric or psychological

DOI: 10.4324/9781003187042-3

problem. However, I had never encountered examples of people hearing voices or seeing visions and viewing them as an accepted part of their life.

Contemporary Western perspectives on voices and visions tend to favour secular, biomedical and psychological explanations for voices and visions (Spittles, 2022). But what about earlier Western perspectives? Simon McCarthy-Jones (2012) maintains that in European traditions, there have been two predominant discourses competing for ascendency through the ages: spiritual explanations and pathological or medical views.

As a junior doctor I had no awareness that there were prominent European historical figures who heard voices and saw visions and found them instructive and helpful. This chapter will offer just a small number of examples from Europe to set the scene for our subsequent exploration of psychiatric perspectives. We turn first to Athens, Greece, for a description of voice-hearing dating back to the fourth century BC, in which the philosopher Plato recounts the explanation given by his teacher Socrates.

Socrates

In 399 BC Socrates found himself at the centre of a trial by jury, accused of heresy and corrupting young minds (Plato, 1993). By this time he was 70. Over several decades he had attracted enemies amongst the ruling class in Athens due to his willingness to scrutinise and publicly criticise the unethical behaviour of a range of public figures.

The court proceedings were witnessed by a 500-strong male jury as well as other members of the public. Plato, his friend and student, was among the onlookers. The words Socrates spoke in his own defence were recalled in detail by Plato and handed down to posterity in the form of a dialogue between Socrates and others present, such as his prosecutor, Meletus. At the end of the trial, the jury found him guilty as charged by a margin of 60 votes. A debate then took place about what would be the appropriate punishment, with the prosecution making a case for the death penalty. Socrates argued on his own behalf that the punishment he deserved was free meals in an exclusive establishment at the expense of the state, explaining that he had been providing an important service to society. Apparently unimpressed with his attitude, the jury condemned him to death by an increased majority of two-thirds.

Socrates stood before the jury one last time. During this speech, he addressed those members who had voted to acquit him, attempting to console them regarding his impending demise. He explained that throughout many years in his life he had heard a prophetic voice which he called his 'divine sign'. He described this voice as his constant companion. He explained that it had opposed him frequently in his life when he was about to take a wrong course of action. The voice had been so particular that it had been known to interrupt him in mid-sentence to correct him. He then revealed that during the final day of his trial, at no point did the voice correct him or argue for any change to his words or actions. It had been such a reliable guide in his life that he was convinced it would always correct him in the case of any error. Therefore, he was sure that his death sentence would turn out to be a blessing. His conclusion was that it was a mistake to assume that death is evil (Plato, 1993).

From this vantage point, over 2,400 years later, what are we to make of Socrates' description? Assuming that Plato's account of what his teacher said is accurate, what was he experiencing? As a psychiatrist, I have been trained to consider a range of possible explanations for a person's perceptual experiences. Socrates, in referring to the voice he heard as his divine sign, clearly believed there was a spiritual explanation for his experience. My training would lead me to consider whether any other causes might be plausible. Could his description fit with a possible psychotic cause? Could there be a psychological explanation for what he described? Was this the voice of his conscience rather than an external perception? Was there any organic brain condition that could result in similar experiences which sound like verbal hallucinations? Could he have been consuming substances which might have accounted for his experiences?

A careful evaluation of a range of alternative diagnoses or explanations is considered integral to good practice of clinical medicine. Such a mindset is critical for recognising non-obvious but potentially harmful or even lethal conditions at an early stage. I would require this from any doctor I am consulting for my own healthcare. As a psychiatrist, whenever I am seeing someone with psychiatric symptoms, such as hearing voices or seeing visions, part of my job is to consider possible medical causes such as temporal lobe epilepsy, or perhaps a brain tumour.

Socrates, as seen through the writings of Plato and others, is commonly regarded as one of the great philosophers (Plato, 1993). He was unrelenting in his quest for self-knowledge and was just as uncompromising in applying rational thought to examining his values and beliefs and those of his contemporaries. Some fellow Athenians also viewed him as odd and eccentric. He walked long distances barefoot and had little interest in money or family life. Instead, he frequented public places, questioning others to assist them to identify the limits of their understanding (Skodlar & Jørgensen, 2013). Some of his beliefs and behaviour may have been viewed as bizarre by his contemporaries. He was reported to stand silent like a statue for hours at a time. This behaviour led Pinel in 1818 to suggest Socrates may have been suffering from catalepsy – a condition described in some people with severe psychotic illnesses in which they may adopt rigid postures. Other writers have suggested he suffered from schizophrenia due to the voices he heard and his odd behaviour (Skodlar & Jørgensen, 2013).

At the same time, there is no evidence from first-hand accounts that Socrates' behaviour was disorganised. He is depicted in Plato's dialogues as highly organised in his arguments, and very rational. While he displayed no fear of death and declined an opportunity to escape his execution, it seems these responses arose from faith in his divine sign and beliefs about the afterlife rather than any psychotic disorder. Socrates certainly saw no conflict between rational thinking and having a belief in signs such as the voice he heard (Skodlar & Jørgensen, 2013).

Contemporary historians and some medical writers have criticised the practice of assigning a retrospective diagnosis to any historical figure (Mitchell, 2011; Muramoto, 2014). They argue that it is impossible to carry out any aspect of a proper medical or psychiatric history or examination, or any other investigation. Therefore, any diagnosis is purely speculative. Furthermore, ethical concerns have been raised about drawing a conclusion about someone's medical or psychiatric state without ever meeting them, having a physician-patient relationship with them or having any chance to seek their consent. In addition, there is concern about conclusions based on narrow medical criteria without taking into account the broad range of other social science literature that is often available. Finally, there is concern about making diagnoses that did not exist at that time (Muramoto, 2014).

If Socrates were to have consulted a physician about his voice-hearing experiences, what would they have concluded? Hippocrates, who was a contemporary of Socrates, was a Greek physician who advocated for careful empirical observation of disease processes and documentation of findings so that these could be passed down to other physicians (Kauffman & McLennan, 2017). He focused on diseases and their relationship with body pathology rather than any beliefs that they might be visited on people by gods or deities. He identified several patterns of mental disorder, including mania (insanity), melancholy (which he maintained was a disorder of black bile) and phrenitis (a form of delirium). Cornelius Celsus was a subsequent Roman writer who translated Greek medical texts into Latin in the first century AD. He noted that hallucinations, presumably including voices and visions, could occur in each of the mental states outlined above in Hippocratic writings (McCarthy-Jones, 2012). So, it's possible that a physician at the time of Socrates could have considered his voice-hearing experiences as a product of his brain rather than emanating from a spiritual source.

Would Socrates' voice-hearing experiences fit contemporary definitions of auditory hallucinations? According to the DSM-5, hallucinations are defined as 'perception-like experiences that occur without an external stimulus'. They are often vivid and clear 'with the full force and impact of normal perceptions' and not under a person's voluntary control (American Psychiatric Association, 2013). According to Plato's account, it is very possible that the voice or voices Socrates heard would have met this definition. The description suggests he heard the voice when his sensorium or state of mind was otherwise clear – another feature of this definition.

However, the DSM-5 definition raises a question about how one might decide that a perception-like experience has no external stimulus. As a clinician, one rule of thumb I could use is that if I can't hear the voice, there must be no external stimulus. On the face of it, this would appear to be common sense. However, in my work with Wiremu, I have had instances when I have seen and heard nothing, but Wiremu is confident that there is a spiritual entity in the room that explains a person's experiences because he can see them too. An example of this is described in Jake's story in Chapter 8. So perhaps common sense in this case is dependent on my beliefs and worldview. As a Western-trained clinician, I have been educated to think about experience in a secular way. I have inherited a tradition of thinking that has been handed down by many generations of medical school teachers and scientists that spiritual experience is not part of what we do. Perhaps these values can be traced back to René Descartes (1596–1650), John Locke (1632–1704) and other philosophers of the Enlightenment age who focused on the importance of reasoned arguments and were determined to emancipate science from the influence of the church.

What about in Socrates' case? I expect Socrates was confident that his 'accustomed sign' had an external divine stimulus. If he could have been asked whether his voices were hallucinations as defined by the DSM-5, my hunch is his response would have been 'no'. Western medical writers who have suggested that Socrates was suffering from schizophrenia or another psychotic condition clearly believed his experiences occurred to him without any external stimulus. Presumably that would exclude any spiritual cause for his experiences from that viewpoint. Other contemporary neuroscientists might argue that his voice could have been an example of 'inner speech'. We will explore this concept more in the next chapter. In either case, there is a tacit secular assumption that is common to Western medical academic writing and thinking. However, what is the basis of this assumption? To what extent is it a function of our worldviews formed from the beliefs we have grown up with in our cultures and the traditions of thinking we have been trained in or come to value?

Wiremu

When I consider Socrates' description of his voice-hearing experiences, my initial response is that they could fit with either spiritual experiences or a brain problem. The fact that he readily accepted the death penalty raises the question of whether he was of sound mind. Many people would ask how a rational person could accept that. If he was being irrational, perhaps that is a sign he had a brain problem or illness. On the other hand, I'm interested in his kōrero (explanation) about death not being an evil thing. That makes sense to me because whether it's today or tomorrow, we all have to die sometime. In weighing up the evidence for a brain problem against details that suggest a spiritual experience, I am inclined to think his voice hearing was spiritual. Socrates was known for his rational thinking. He was a philosopher and a critical thinker. He was convinced his experience was a divine voice. It had been with him for many years. Over the years, it had proved itself through repeated helpful guidance. I am familiar with my own voices that have had a similar guiding role that I can trust. They haven't done me wrong yet, so I trust them in situations of uncertainty.

Allister

In order to reflect further on different cultural meanings of voices, visions and hallucinations in relation to Socrates' experiences, I would like to digress briefly. In 1993, when I was based at the Family Centre, the social services agency I referred to in Chapter 1, the centre carried out a unique research project. The Family Centre research team were undertaking fono or group research with separate male and female Samoan elder groups, service providers and people with lived experience of mental distress. These fono took place in the Samoan language with fa'asamoa (Samoan worldviews) protocols. The venue was the front room of the Family Centre. In the preparation for this study, known as Ole Taeao Afua, elders advised the research team that the question 'What would it take to develop a mental health service that was appropriate for Samoan people?' was difficult to address in a fa'asamoa context without first establishing the nature of a Samoan sense of self (Tamasese et al., 2005). Elders in the study described a Samoan sense of self as relational and spiritual.

Having grown up in a Palagi (New Zealand European) community with strong values of individuality and secular ways of doing things, I found it hard to get my head around the significance of that distinction. Yet participants in this study declared that in fa'asamoa, spirituality and mental well-being were so closely intertwined that any mental health intervention that didn't take spirituality into account was unlikely to be effective or relevant for Samoan people. The elder women's group provided narratives explaining the nature of spirituality that highlighted perceptual experiences that might be considered unusual from a Western perspective (Tamasese et al., 1997). For example, it described instances from the 1950s in which an elderly woman, known to be alive in her village on Upolu, was seen on a number of occasions by multiple family members in a village in Savai'i, a considerable distance away over ocean and land. It was implied that her spirit must have travelled between the islands without usual means of transport (Tamasese et al., 1997). Such spiritual occurrences were considered by these Samoan participants to be part of the continuum of human experience.

During a session on culture and psychiatry that I teach to medical students, I describe this research and the conclusions from the elders about the relational and spiritual nature of the Samoan self. I then ask the students to place themselves on an imaginary line from one end of our seminar room to the other, with an individual self at one end and a relational self at the other, and invite them to comment on why they placed themselves there. I then ask them to do the same again, but this time with a spiritual sense of self at one end and a secular sense of self at the other. I again invite students to comment on where they positioned themselves this time. This always leads to interesting conversations.

In thinking about the DSM-5 definition of hallucination and Socrates' description of his voice, where would you place yourself on that imaginary line, with a spiritual sense of self at one end and a secular sense of self at the other? Spiritual in this context can mean whatever you prefer it to mean. Secular I define as 'nonspiritual'. What I have noticed is that medical schools, hospitals and mainstream mental health services in Aotearoa have tacit secular assumptions. By that I mean spiritual practices are generally not accepted as part of what we do. For example, it would be considered strange and inappropriate if a consultant physician or surgeon was to offer to pray for a patient or their family on a ward round. Similarly, from a Pākehā or Western perspective, with values favouring individual rights to your own form of religious expression, starting my teaching session with a prayer would be viewed as impinging on the individual rights of students in the group to have their own spiritual or secular values and practices. I notice that it is the opposite in the Māori and Pacific settings I work in. Elders such as kaumātua will frequently start a session with a karakia or prayer because that is the appropriate kawa (protocol) for our service. The tacit assumption is spiritual and relational; it is assumed that it is necessary to take care of the spiritual wellbeing of the whole group rather than leaving it for individuals to do it themselves if they choose to.

Returning to the voice of Socrates, it seems he had a clear spiritual assumption about the origin of this voice. What strikes me here was the relationship between Socrates and his 'accustomed sign'. He completely trusted its judgement. Given that he was such a critical and independent thinker in many areas of his life, it is apparent that he had faith in the guidance of his voice, even regarding his death. I wonder how he arrived at this sense of trust. Perhaps he had so many experiences of the voice's guidance over decades that he trusted what the voice said implicitly.

In the rest of this chapter, we will look at the experiences and writings of three women: Hildegard of Bingen, Joan of Arc and St Teresa of Ávila; and one man, Thomas Aquinas. They span 500 years, from the early 1100s to the late 1500s. Following this, we will examine descriptions from children of their voice-hearing and visions: firstly, from a boy in Victorian England who described his own experiences in everyday life, then to the experiences of three children shortly after the Portuguese revolution in 1910. Wiremu will give his response following each of these narratives.

Hildegard of Bingen

Hildegard of Bingen (1098–1179) was a German saint who had her first vision before the age of five. She later recalled seeing such 'a great light that my soul quaked' (Flanagan, 1998). Hildegard explained, 'When I was filled with this vision, I said many things that were strange to the hearers' (Flanagan, 1998). After she began to realise that others didn't see the things she was seeing, she learned to hide her experiences from those around her.

Hildegard continued to have striking visions filled with light in her early adult years, but it was not until she was 42 that she had an experience that transformed her outlook. This time she described seeing a 'fiery light' which entered her and set her mind, heart and chest 'afire like a flame – yet not burning but warming, as the sun warms an object on which it sheds its rays' (Newman, 1985). She described that she suddenly had a clear understanding of scriptures that she wasn't able to read and of many visions from throughout her life. Around this time, she heard a voice 'from heaven' telling her, 'Write what you see and hear' (Flanagan, 1998). From this time, Hildegard began to tell others about her visions and her new understanding of sacred texts. She began to compose songs and chants despite having had no previous training. She published books that outlined her visions and her interpretations of them in great detail (Foxhall, 2014). Later in life, she continued to report seeing her 'living light' at certain times, always associated with a feeling of joy (Flanagan, 1998).

Hildegard clearly viewed her experiences as having profound spiritual significance. However, medical writers have interpreted her visions differently. In 1917, a medical historian called Charles Singer published an article which examined the detail of some of her illustrations of her visions and concluded that she may have been experiencing migraine auras (Foxhall, 2014). For example, in one of Hildegard's pictures, Singer interpreted features that resembled castle ramparts as 'fortification spectra', a feature of migraine aura in which zigzag lines appear across someone's visual field. He interpreted other illustrations as depictions of scintillating scotoma, which are one or more blind spots flickering between light and dark, a characteristic feature of aura for many migraine sufferers (Viana et al., 2019). As a result, medical writers have dismissed Hildegard's spiritual interpretations of her experiences and concluded that her voices and visions can be explained in purely neurological terms (Foxhall, 2014). After reading about this, I was curious to seek Wiremu's view about Hildegard's experiences and the medical interpretation of them.

Wiremu

I'm interested in Hildegard's description of having to hide her experiences from others after she realised that no one else was seeing the light she could see. In Chapter 9, I explain 'noho puku', which is when people go silent and sit on their experience. They may choose not to speak about it because they believe no one will understand. It sounds like Hildegard kept most of her experiences to herself until her early 40s. When I hear her later description of her experience of the 'living light', and how her songs and music came to her, it seems likely to me that she was very familiar with spiritual experiences. When she said, 'I compose no other words than those I hear and I set them forth in unpolished Latin, just as I hear them in the vision' (Newman, 1985), that sounds like a wairua download to me. Matekite (spiritual awareness) is linked to creativity. For many years I was a musician and would compose songs for my band. Sometimes I still have experiences where a song will come to me very early in the morning. It may even wake me up and I think, 'I've got to get a pen.' One song that I received in this way was *Tōtara Tree*. The night before I heard that a kaumātua who had been a big support for our youth programme in Gisborne had passed away. At 3 AM I woke up and climbed out of my van. Standing right there in front of me was a majestic tōtara tree. I grabbed my guitar out of the van and sat under the tree. The tune and the words for the song came to me effortlessly. It felt like a wairua download.

With regards to the migraine hypothesis, I expect a doctor would need to be able to ask Hildegard about her symptoms to clarify that matter. However, even if she did have migraines, that doesn't preclude her from having spiritual experiences as well. Anything that alters the mind could also, in some people, open up a doorway. It's possible that migraines could have helped unlock a connection to the other side. This can have positive or negative effects. You only need to listen to the songs she wrote to know that she had something pretty positive coming through.

Allister

While medical historians have given their 20th-century perspectives on Hildegard's experiences, how would medical thinkers and theologians who came soon after her have viewed her experiences? The next prominent figure we turn to gives us an insight into one line of mainstream church thinking at that time in Europe.

Thomas Aquinas

Thomas Aquinas (1225–1274), an Italian theologian and Dominican priest, wrote about a range of causes for voices. He argued that voice-hearing could be due to natural reasons and highlighted the use of herbal preparations that might cause people to hear voices (McCarthy-Jones, 2012). He also noted that voice-hearing could be caused by physiological changes, or by people thinking the experiences they had created in their imagination were real. A further cause he outlined was madness or a disease of the body.

As a result, Thomas maintained that some people who called themselves prophets were not prophets. He also outlined a range of possible supernatural causes of voice-hearing, and believed voices were one way of receiving divine revelation (McCarthy-Jones, 2012).

Joan of Arc

Joan of Arc (1412–1431) was born in the village of Domrémy in the north of what is now France. At this time French communities had been devastated by a long-running conflict with the English Crown, known as the Hundred Years' War. Morale was low due to a series of French defeats over three decades. Joan had several older siblings, and her parents were farmers. Around the time the war reached Domrémy, Joan had her first experiences of visions and voices. Most of the detail documented about her experiences are from transcripts from her heresy trial a few years later (Murray, 1902).

At her trial, Joan declared that she first heard a voice when she was 13. At around midday on a summer's day, she heard a voice coming from her right side, which she realised was the direction of the village church. On this and subsequent occasions, Joan recalled that the voice was accompanied by a particular light. This voice later identified itself to her as St Michael, and she described how on some occasions she could see him with her physical eyes 'as well as I see you' (Murray, 1902). Although initially frightened, over time Joan came to believe that her experiences had been sent by God. At other times she reported seeing and hearing two female saints, Catherine and Margaret, who provided her with frequent guidance and counsel.

About three years later, Joan's voices began to insist she go to France to break the siege of the City of Orléans. The voices told her to travel to the town of Vaucouleurs, some 20 kilometres away, where she should approach the captain of the guard, Robert de Baudricourt (Murray, 1902). She said she managed to persuade her uncle to take her to Vaucouleurs, and when she was there, her voices helped her identify Baudricourt. As predicted by Joan's voices, Baudricourt twice refused to meet her before finally agreeing to meet. Even then, he rejected her request for help and sent her away. At the behest of her voices, Joan persisted. A local duke intervened, and Baudricourt agreed to help her (Castor, 2014). Joan travelled on horseback over 500 kilometres through enemy territory, dressed in men's clothing and accompanied by an armed escort. Her quest was an audience with Charles, the dauphin (heir to the French throne), who was aged about 26 at the time.

When Charles was growing up, his father, King Charles VI, had been severely afflicted by a psychotic illness. Although initially popular, King Charles VI developed persecutory delusions during a military campaign in his early 20s and fatally attacked some of his own knights (Sinha, 2021). For the rest of his life, King Charles VI suffered from recurring episodes of psychosis, during which he had a prominent delusional belief that he was made of glass. His illness contributed to a period of compromised leadership in France (Castor, 2014).

As a result of his father's illness, Charles junior would have had plenty of life experiences to help him recognise if Joan was suffering from a mental illness, despite the attraction of her claim to hear divine voices that promised to help him regain his kingdom. His situation was desperate. The dauphin and his court had been forced to retreat to a centre south of Paris while large areas of the north of France were occupied by English military and their French allies. According to the historian Helen Castor (2014), it was common knowledge at this time that people of sound mind could hear voices and see visions. It was assumed that these experiences could bring communication from divine or evil sources.

Charles decided that he would ask a council of the most senior clergy and theologians available to him to meet with Joan and investigate her claims to divine guidance. After three weeks of interrogation and testing, they concluded she was of sound character and her claims might be authentic. She was brought to meet Charles, but as a further test she was first introduced to two different officials, each disguised as Charles. In both cases, guided by her voices, she recognised that she was being deceived. Joan subsequently correctly identified Charles when she was finally in his presence. In addition, she offered Charles a further way to test her guidance. She explained to him that her voices had revealed to her the exact location of a sword hidden in St Catherine's church in the distant town of Sainte-Catherine-de-Fierbois. The instructions she gave to Charles correctly identified the exact location of this sword buried behind the altar of the church. When Charles' emissary returned with this sword and explained how it had been recovered, and the surprise of the local clergy, he was further persuaded that her voices and visions could be authentic.

The final test suggested by the council of clergy was a practical one. During her interrogation, Joan had claimed that she had been sent to break the siege at Orléans. Morale was then so low in France that the situation at

Orléans was considered hopeless. The clergy suggested to Charles that he give her a limited company of troops to proceed to Orléans and test whether her claims to divine inspiration could be proven by action and results (Castor, 2014).

During her later heresy trial, Joan said she had told Charles that she would be injured in the neck at Orléans, but that she would be able to continue her 'work' (Murray, 1902). She said this event had been predicted by 'the voices of my two saints'. Joan described being hit by a crossbolt in the neck during the attack on a bridge fortress at Orléans but explained she had been given 'great comfort from St Catherine' and had recovered rapidly (Murray, 1902). Twenty-five years later, when Joan was retried and her previous conviction of heresy was overturned, evidence included a letter from a Flemish diplomat which outlined her prediction of this injury. The letter was dated 15 days before she sustained the injury (Wayman, 1957).

The history of Joan's astonishing leadership during the battle of Orléans is well known. The siege was broken within nine days of her arrival, after just four days of fighting. Over the following eight months Joan continued to inspire French forces in a series of battles, and the English armies and their allies sustained a sequence of heavy defeats. However, following a truce, in May 1430 Joan was captured and handed over to the English. In January 1431, at the age of 19, she was put on trial on charges of heresy. The court was composed of church officials who supported the English king, Henry VI. The charges included an allegation that Joan had blasphemed by wearing men's clothing. Despite the sham nature of the court process, in which it was clear that her eventual execution was a foregone conclusion, significant efforts were made to carefully record all Joan's statements made in the courtroom, including her responses under cross-examination. This resulted in a unique record of her own views about her experiences of voices and visions. Even though these transcripts were ultimately used to justify her condemnation and execution, her composure under provoking interrogation and her loyalty to the counsel of her voices shone through.

What might we make of Joan's experiences of visions and voices from our contemporary perspective? Is it possible that she was correct, and her voices emanated from a divine Source? Are there any other plausible explanations? From the viewpoints of 19th- and 20th-century medicine, writers have suggested several brain problems that might account for her experiences, including psychosis and epilepsy (Schildkrout, 2017). Her descriptions suggest her symptoms were episodic and her thinking was quite clear at other times, which could be consistent with epilepsy. Some writers have suggested her positive feeling at the time of seeing her visions and hearing the voices could be due to ecstatic auras, again due to a type of seizure. Others have suggested that her visions associated with church bells ringing could have been explained by a type of epilepsy known as reflex epilepsy.

In reading the detail of Joan's exploits, it strikes me that if a person's symptoms of schizophrenia or epilepsy could confer on them the ability to predict one's own future injury in battle, or know the site of a buried sword, or inspire demoralised troops, then perhaps we have underestimated these conditions. As I explained earlier in this chapter, I am in favour of medical perspectives that help us think critically about possible medical causes for a person's experiences. At the same time, I don't think it serves us well to completely dismiss spiritual worldviews. I wish I had the opportunity to ask each of these medical writers where they would have placed themselves on the continuum between a secular sense of self and a spiritual sense of self. My hunch is that their perspectives may reflect secular worldviews.

Wiremu

When I was young, Catholic priests used to visit Tiniroto and host retreats for local kids. I went a few times because they had nice biscuits. I remember they had flipcharts with beautiful pictures of saints, including Joan of Arc and St Teresa. They would tell stories about their lives. Just like the pūrākau (narratives) that my kuia (female elder) told us, these stories would bring them to life in my imagination.

Joan of Arc became a heroine of mine. I have little doubt that she was both a matekite (someone with spiritual awareness) and a matakite (someone with foresight). She was a visionary. She not only heard voices and saw visions, but they gave her insight into what she was meant to be doing. They guided her. She demonstrated that, in a few instances, she could see the future, which is by my definition the gift of matakite. I have met many people who describe similar experiences of hearing voices and seeing apparitions. They haven't gone out to fight any battles, but they have identified something that later came to pass and that they were unlikely to have been able to predict by chance.

In Chapter 2 I recounted stories about Toiroa, Te Kooti and Wiremu Ratana, who were our own prophets, our own seers, and who foretold events that later came to pass. It seems to me Joan of Arc had a similar gift. She was connected to her divine Source. Her awareness of the sword's whereabouts and her future injury are evidence for her matakite. Experiences like hers are familiar to me and are known in te ao Māori (the Māori world). In my view, the response from the church in which she was burnt at the stake is also typical of church responses to matekite individuals in many times and places. There was a missed opportunity here to encourage her to develop her gift further as a matekite and as a leader.

This kōrero also raises an interesting question about good and evil. The question that people often ask about a spiritual presence is whether it is a good spirit or a bad spirit. So, if we ask this question about Joan of Arc and her voices and visions, what can we conclude? Were the voices and visions she heard good or bad spirits? History would tell us that she won a number of battles, and this suggests that the guidance she received was helpful: that these entities were on her side. It strikes me that the rigged trial in which she was wrongly condemned to death was an evil process. However, sometimes I think that making distinctions between good and evil can depend on which side you are on. From the point of view of the slain English soldiers, were these entities good or evil? And during the trial of Joan, men wearing frocks were judging Joan for wearing trousers without a penis. Even more than her alleged crossdressing, they were judging her on whether she had the authority to hear voices or see visions without their say-so. It was all about power and control. It makes sense to me that people would say this was an evil process. On the other hand, as a result of the process of this trial, we have a detailed account of Joan's kōrero about her experiences which we can learn from. So, something good has come out of this for us centuries later.

Allister

St Teresa of Ávila

About 100 years after Joan, in 1534, Saint Teresa of Ávila (1515–1582) entered the Carmelite Convent at Ávila in central Spain at the age of 20, following a long period of illness (Saint Teresa, 1957). This Catholic order was focused on silent contemplative practices.

As a young nun, Teresa received visitors to the convent and engaged in extended conversations with them, as was common practice. One day, in the midst of a discussion she was enjoying with a visitor, Teresa suddenly saw a vision of Christ looking directly at her, with a 'most severe' expression on his face (Saint Teresa, 1957). She described seeing this image with the eyes of her soul 'much more clearly than I could ever have seen Him with the eyes of the body'. She felt 'astonished and disturbed', and the experience remained very vivid for her 26 years later. Her interpretation was that God was warning her away from frivolous talk and steering her towards solitude and contemplation.

During periods of meditation and prayer, Teresa would hear 'locutions' or internal voices which she viewed as an ordinary part of her life (Saint Teresa, 1957). Over time she came to the conclusion that some of the voices she heard were from God. She described these voices as distinct, not heard by the physical ear, and said they 'had to be listened to' (McCarthy-Jones, 2012). These voices corrected her if she erred and gave her 'both counsel and relief'. They made prophecies of future events, many of which she reported as being fulfilled, sometimes several years later

(Saint Teresa, 1957). In addition to her voice-hearing experiences, Teresa had visions of deceased monks and saints from previous generations.

It is clear from Teresa's writing that she experienced moments of worry and doubt throughout her life. In contrast, her visions and voice-hearing experiences were often accompanied by intense positive emotional and spiritual feelings, such as one incident when she reported feeling a 'state of union' with God (Saint Teresa, 1957).

Teresa wrote about features of voices which she believed indicated they came from God. One was the sense of authority they conveyed. Another was a deep feeling of tranquillity they brought to the hearer, and the way the words remained easily recalled for a long time (Saint Teresa, 1957).

Teresa supported early medical interpretations of voices, commenting that often voices could be a sign of unwellness, especially in people who were affected by 'real melancholy'. At the same time, she had political reasons for supporting medical interpretations of these experiences. Simon McCarthy-Jones (2012) has pointed out that by labelling some of her fellow sisters as sick, she was able to save them from death during the Spanish Inquisition.

Wiremu

It seems to me that the voices and visions that St Teresa described could be consistent with her being a matekite. Without meaning to be disrespectful, I have a question about her story about seeing Christ giving her a stern look. I have no problem with the possibility that Christ could communicate with her that way. However, I'm curious to know what led her to conclude it was Christ she saw. Given that he didn't identify himself verbally, what was it about his appearance that told her this? What does Christ look like? What kind of face would he have when he is stern? Unless she had seen a photograph of Christ, how would she know what he looked like? I'm not questioning that she could have seen Jesus or God: just pointing out that her conclusion is her interpretation based on the clues she has noticed in her experience. I would also say that as an experienced matekite, she is the one who is best placed to decide who it was she saw.

Allister

We now move on to examples of voices and visions, as reported by a child in Victorian England.

The Boy Who Saw True

The Boy Who Saw True is the title of a book that consists of diary entries from a young boy who grew up in England in the mid-1880s, written when he was seven to ten years old (S.L., 1953). At the time he wrote his diary, it appears he had no intention that anyone would read it. Many years later, at the end of his life, his wife persuaded him to have it published. He reluctantly agreed on the condition that it be available only after his death, hence its publication in 1953. To protect the privacy of people in his life, it was published anonymously and all names and some other details in the diary were changed.

The diary entries are notable for their candour and naivety as the boy describes many aspects of his life, his feelings and reactions to events. At some point, it becomes apparent that he is seeing things that others are not. One day his father arrives home from work, and the boy is surprised to see his uncle sitting in his father's chair in the living room. He shouts out in alarm when his father, unaware of the uncle's presence, sits down on top of him. When he explains his concern, his father scolds him for telling lies, and insists that this uncle has been dead for many months (S.L., 1953).

He also writes about seeing a figure with long brown hair and blue eyes standing at the end of his bed, smiling at him. He comments that seeing this man makes him feel very happy and concludes that it must be Jesus. He later asks his mother if she also sees Jesus, and she becomes angry and accuses him of making up stories. He describes seeing lights around people, and over time he compares the 'lovely lights' he sees around 'Jesus' with the 'dirty lights' he sees around an aunty who makes him feel distinctly uncomfortable. Months later he sees something crab-like 'sticking' to an older woman which he describes as 'horrid'. The author's notes from late in his life mention that this person died from cancer 18 months later. Her illness did not appear to be obvious to others at the time.

It is apparent from diary entries that he is becoming aware that he is seeing people and things that others can't see. His older sister teases him about his 'lies', and he stops revealing his experiences to others. Meanwhile, his mother arranges to get his eyes checked. Later he sees a doctor who asks him lots of questions, including whether he hears noises when nobody is in the room. At a follow-up appointment, the doctor is apparently nonplussed when the boy sees an older woman in the room. His description closely resembles the doctor's deceased mother, whom the boy has never met (S.L., 1953).

Wiremu

When I reflect on the diary notes by the boy from Victorian England, I notice that at a young age he was told to stop telling lies when he spoke to his parents about his experiences. In fact, his own view from late in his life was that his mother had assumed he was either 'an incorrigible little liar' or 'heading for the lunatic asylum' (S.L., 1953). He concludes as an old man that he has been clairvoyant all his life and does not describe any problems with mental illness. Certainly, his experiences as a boy sound like normal spiritual voices and visions to me. I remember at his age I was often puzzled by similar experiences. I was fortunate that I could go to my kuia. She knew that I had a gift and she explained it to me.

However, others around me, such as my whāngai (adoptive) siblings, often thought I was making things up or being smart to get attention.

If young people with these gifts are not supported and believed, they may internalise their confusion. Their minds can become conflicted. If they have no way to share this experience safely and no one to explain what they are going through, over time they may start to believe they are losing their mind. The stress of this could contribute to them becoming mentally unwell. In Chapter 9, I return to this matter and outline some approaches to manaaki (support) young people who are matekite, like this boy.

For example, it is really important to help them understand what's happening and to shed some light on what they are going through. During the interaction when the boy sees the woman, it dawns on the doctor that this old lady bears an uncanny resemblance to his own deceased mother. This kind of situation can jolt people into a new understanding. Such moments can lead to a breakthrough for people in my mahi (work). I expect the boy's doctor was racking his brains thinking, 'How the heck did this boy know what my mother looked like?' He was very likely wondering if there was another explanation. For example, had he accidently left a photo of his mother lying around somewhere?

With regard to the boy's vision of the crab on the woman who had cancer, this is an example of matekite: seeing sickness in someone. That was a tohu, a sign. He was seeing a sign of sickness on her. Sometimes I have seen signs like that. For example, in the past I would sometimes see a bird's beak on part of a person's body, such as their head. Often that was a sign that that person had pain in that part of their body, such as severe headaches or migraines, or pain in their shoulder joint if the bird's beak was on their shoulder. All I would see was the beak, not the bird's head or eyes. Seeing that crab could also be an example of foresight, or matakite. You could say that he is able to see ahead that this woman has this particular illness. It has that predictive quality. The boy wrote his diary in the 1880s, suggesting to me that wairua hasn't changed much. This boy was a seer. It's not just a Māori thing.

When the boy talked about seeing lights around people, he was referring to seeing their mauri. Some people might call that an aura. I often see colours around people. It's the mauri that gives us life. That is the physical manifestation of wairua. Some healers use that ability to detect spiritual health problems by looking at the person's mauri. For example, Kapi Adams and Te Awhina Riwaka were both renowned tohunga (Māori healers) who worked like this. There are many different matekite gifts that can contribute to healing.

If you can see someone's mauri and it's burning brightly, that indicates that they are likely to be spiritually healthy and most often physically well. When you see someone's mauri looking diminished, that can indicate that the person is physically unwell. When a person dies, then by definition their mauri is extinguished. After death, the wairua still exists, but the mauri, the life force, is gone. The kōrero is that the creator breathed into our nostrils, and we became living beings. The breath given by the Creator is the mauri. My mauri is a contract between Te Kaihanga and myself. When the mauri is extinguished, the wairua hasn't died, but the fuel that runs the vehicle has gone. Wairua carries on.

Allister

The Children of Fátima

The Portuguese revolution of 1910 ended a centuries-old monarchy and replaced it with a republic which sought to suppress the influence of the Catholic Church and promote science and rationalism. Around this time, Lúcia dos Santos (1907–2005) was born in the small village of Aljustrel, 130 kilometres north of Lisbon (dos Santos, 2007). She was the youngest of her seven siblings, and her family farmed land they owned near the village. At the age of seven, Lúcia became responsible for tending the family's flock of sheep during the day, as was the local custom.

The following year, 1915, she and two other companions climbed up to a clearing on the eastern slope of a hill near their village, above a glade of olive and holm oak trees. Lúcia suggested they pray. As they did so, Lúcia saw a figure hovering in the air in front of them above the trees (dos Santos, 2007). On that first occasion she described it as being like a statue made of snow that the sun had made appear to be transparent. It disappeared just as they finished their prayers. She decided not to mention it to her family, but her companions told their siblings and before long word got back to her mother, who questioned her about it. Lúcia recalled that she told her mother that she didn't know what it might be, but it resembled a person wrapped up in a sheet, meaning that she couldn't make out any details. She recalled that her mother made a 'gesture of disgust' and dismissed her experience as 'childish nonsense' (dos Santos, 2007). Over the following months her siblings teased her about seeing people wrapped up in sheets. Later that year the same figure appeared twice more in the same place.

In 1916, Lúcia was tending sheep on the same hill with her two cousins, Jacinta Marto (1910–1920) and Francisco Marto (1908–1919), when they saw what Lúcia said was the same figure she had seen the year before. She later wrote that the figure looked male, aged perhaps 14 or 15. It was 'whiter than snow' and 'transparent as crystal' when the sun was shining behind it (dos Santos, 2007). She described it as very beautiful. This figure was initially suspended above the trees as before, but then came down and knelt beside them and spoke, saying, 'Do not be afraid, I am the angel of peace. Pray with me.' After her previous experience, she warned Jacinta and Francisco against telling anyone about it. On two further occasions that year the same figure visited the three cousins at the same spot on that hillside.

At around midday on 13 May 1917, Lúcia and her cousins were on the same hillside when they saw a woman appear before them just a few feet away. Lúcia described her as dressed all in white and radiating light, 'more brilliant than the sun' (dos Santos, 2007). The woman spoke to them saying, 'Do not be afraid. I will do you no harm.' Although all three of them could see her, only Lúcia and Jacinta could hear her speak. Lúcia then asked her where she was from and she replied, 'from heaven'. When Lúcia asked her what she wanted, the woman said she had come to ask them to return on the 13th day of each month, to the same spot, at the same time, for six months in a row. She said she would reveal her identity in due course and explain what she wanted of them.

Lúcia asked her whether they would go to heaven, and she received specific answers for each of them. The woman then asked them if they would offer themselves to God, and bear suffering for God. When they said they were willing, the woman told them, 'Then you are going to have much to suffer, but the grace of God will be your comfort.' Lúcia reported that as she finished that statement, the woman opened her hands and an intense light streamed towards them and 'penetrated our hearts and the innermost depths of our souls'. They then fell to their knees and prayed. Finally, the woman told them, 'Pray the rosary every day in order to obtain peace for the world and the end of the war.' Then the figure rose and disappeared.

After Jacinta told her family about the visitation, the parish priest interviewed the three children. Meanwhile, Lúcia's mother wanted her to say the whole thing was a lie.

On 13 June the three children returned to the same spot on the hillside and the woman appeared to them again. This time she told Lúcia that she needed to learn to read. When Lúcia asked if the three of them would be going to heaven, the woman responded that she would be taking Jacinta and Francisco there soon, but Lúcia would have to wait. Each time the children returned to the same hillside location on the 13th of the month, they witnessed a visit from the same figure. The exception was 13 August, at which time the local government administrator arranged for them to be detained in a prison cell for 48 hours (dos Santos, 2007). He did this because huge crowds of people had begun to accompany the children and he was perhaps concerned that the situation was disrupting the secular values of the government. The administrator interrogated and threatened the children, but their account didn't change. By late September, two officials from the Catholic Church separately interviewed each of the children about their experiences in detail. Their accounts were very similar, except that Francisco could only describe what he had seen as he had not heard the woman speak.

The final time the figure appeared to the children was 13 October 1917 (dos Santos, 2007). Francisco died from Spanish influenza in 1919 and Jacinta died the following year. Lúcia became a nun and continued to report having similar visions later in her life. There is no indication in accounts of her life that she suffered from any physical or mental illnesses that might have accounted for such experiences. She died aged 97 in 2005.

Wiremu

When the Catholic priests used to visit Tiniroto, they showed us a beautiful picture of those three children sitting in front of the statue of what they called the Lady of the Sacred Heart. The Catholic Church teaches that the woman who appeared to those children was the Virgin Mary, who in Portugal is known as Fátima.

How can we understand what happened to those children on that hillside in Portugal? Did they make it up to get attention? Was it a propaganda exercise for the Catholic Church? There are a number of details in this story that I find interesting. One aspect is that they each had their own experience, but they all could see an apparition of a woman. And they saw her at the same time. The two girls also heard her speak and gave separate accounts describing her speaking some of the same words. Therefore, these three children had a shared experience. In my view, it's much harder to argue that an experience is a figment of someone's imagination when it's a shared experience. You can't convince me that all three of them were hallucinating or delusional at the same time.

Lúcia, the eldest of the three, realised that talking about this experience would make her mother angry and she would get told off. Therefore, she tried to persuade the other two not to tell anyone. This doesn't sound like someone making up a story to get attention. She was already a very religious child and was very particular about telling the truth. Even though her mother was horrified, and local government officials imprisoned the children to try to suppress the story, hundreds of people were interested and came to believe it really had happened. That doesn't prove it was true, but it does suggest that their shared vision was accepted by local people as consistent with commonly held religious beliefs. The local priest who first interviewed the children was quite sceptical. That's understandable, as the priest's credibility would have been on the line. Later on, senior church people put their dresses on and came to check it out. After a thorough interrogation of these tamariki (children), they concluded that each of the children had seen the apparition.

To further address this question of whether this story was true or made up, I like to return to that kōrero, 'mā te hua ka kitea'. The best way I can think of to discern what's going on here is to judge it by the fruit. What has come of these events? Over the following years, the church built a shrine there. In the more than 100 years since, millions of people have visited that place on pilgrimage. People go to Fátima for healing and there are many stories of people being healed. That's the fruit. If these children made up the story, you would soon find out because no-one would be affected. Mind you, we must also take into account the role of faith here. I often say you only need 1 percent faith to get 100 percent return. Healing can happen if you believe in yourself and believe you can be healed. That 1 percent of walking or travelling to that place could be very significant in contributing to those healing outcomes.

Allister

In this chapter we have recounted examples of visions and voice-hearing experiences reported by women, men and children living in Greece, Germany, France, Spain, England and Portugal over a period of almost 2,500 years. In most of these cases, the cultural context of their experiences included notions of spirituality that accepted some people might be able to perceive voices or visions from God, gods or others. It was commonly viewed that such perceptions might represent messages communicated to them to help, hinder or even harm them. Throughout these years in European culture there have been medical commentators who would argue that such experiences may be caused by body or brain problems such as epilepsy, tertiary syphilis, migraines, brain infections or psychological problems. In the next chapter we will examine the history of such psychiatric conceptions of voices and visions in more detail, as well as contemporary psychological and psychiatric understandings.

Although some neurologists have believed that Hildegard of Bingen may have been suffering from migraines, I expect most psychiatrists reading the stories in this chapter will not jump to the conclusion that the protagonists were suffering from a psychiatric illness. Contemporary definitions of psychiatric disorders such as in DSM-5 stipulate that in order for a person's symptoms to meet criteria for a particular mental disorder, they must be experiencing clinically significant distress and impairment in social, occupational or other areas of functioning in their lives. I would suggest that this criterion would not be met by anyone whose story appears in this chapter.

A different matter relates to the question of whether there is intellectual and academic space in psychiatry to consider spiritual perspectives in mental health, for instance those of Wiremu or healing practitioners from diverse cultures. In the late 1800s and early 1900s in Europe, the perspectives of leading psychiatrists reacting to spiritualist interpretations of the meanings of voices and visions became increasingly biomedical. We will discuss this further in the next chapter.

Given the exercise that I explained earlier in the chapter, with the line from a spiritual sense of self at one end to a secular sense of self at the other, I invite you to take a moment to reflect on where you may have placed yourself on that line, and then your responses to the stories in this chapter. Whether we see ourselves as having more of a spiritual sense of self, a secular sense of self or somewhere in between may contribute to our openness to considering whether the perceptual experiences of others could represent spiritual experiences.

Wiremu

Writing about the experiences of European saints, sages and tamariki is another kūaha. It offers a doorway to different perspectives. Each of those whose stories are contained in this chapter believed that their experiences were spiritual in nature. In most of these cases, medical writers have suggested medical conditions to explain their experiences as due to brain problems. However, in their cultural context, they were accepted as spiritual by many people. Spirituality is not just a Māori thing. People from across the world describe similar experiences. We may view our own wairua as unique and different, but I think there are also fundamental aspects that are shared between our cultures. We are all spiritual beings. That's what I conclude from these stories.

4 Voices and Visions in Psychiatry

Allister Bush and Wiremu NiaNia

Allister

Introduction

In Chapter 1, Wiremu explained the Māori title of this book, *Ngā Kūaha,* which refers to doorways or entranceways. He described that a kūaha could be an 'entranceway into a knowledge space'. In this chapter we will look through a number of 'doorways of understanding' into Western knowledge spaces about what happens when people hear voices and see visions.

Voices and visions are difficult to measure, access and study. In the last 200 years, brain and mind researchers have examined voices and visions from myriad points of view. I have selected research findings, theories and perspectives that I consider influential in shaping collective understandings about voices and visions in psychiatry and psychology. Wiremu offers his responses to a number of these viewpoints.

First, we will turn to contemporary definitions of hallucinations and then look at how voices and visions were understood by several historical figures in psychiatry and psychology. Next, we will examine theories in neuroscience about the causes of hallucinations.

Hallucinations in psychiatry have often been associated with severe psychiatric conditions. These have included diagnoses such as schizophrenia, mood problems such as severe depression and mania, and complex psychological trauma. They may also arise due to people's use of certain substances or from medical conditions affecting the brain. We will look at a number of these conditions and their relevance to understanding voices and visions.

For some people, hearing voices and seeing visions may have nothing to do with any mental health condition. Later in the chapter we will turn to research addressing spiritual interpretations of voices and visions and examine perspectives on the place of spirituality in psychiatric practice.

DOI: 10.4324/9781003187042-4

Current Definitions of Hallucinations

Definitions of hallucinations have not changed significantly since my psychiatry training in the 1990s. Hallucinations are defined as sensory perceptions that do not originate from a stimulus in the outside world and are 'unbidden' (Waters et al., 2016). They are experienced when awake, which rules out dreams. Most definitions require hallucinations to have the properties of real perceptions, such as a compelling sense of reality. For visual hallucinations this can include the requirement that they are perceived to be in external space (Waters et al., 2014).

An important question is how the definition of hallucination can help us identify whether a person's voices or visions are a sign of a mental health problem. False perceptions that people have when going to sleep (hypnagogic) or waking up (hypnopompic) are not considered pathological. Nor are transient voices or visions, such as hearing one or two words or experiencing a vision on a few occasions only. As defined in the DSM-5, hallucinations could also be a normal part of a person's religious experience (American Psychiatric Association, 2013). Hallucinations alone, without other evidence of psychotic symptoms such as delusions (fixed false beliefs), are not enough to meet the criteria for a diagnosis of schizophrenia or other psychotic disorder.

A critical part of diagnostic criteria for all mental health conditions relates to impairment. The symptoms the person is experiencing need to have a major negative impact on their life, affecting work, interpersonal relationships and selfcare. Voices and visions that are not disturbing a person or interfering with their life, and aren't associated with other distressing mental health symptoms, do not constitute a mental disorder.

Some views within psychiatry have changed in recent decades. In my training in psychiatry, I was taught it was possible to distinguish between voices heard by people with a psychotic disorder and by people who have experienced trauma. Psychotic voices were considered 'true' hallucinations and were heard external to the person, as if perceived by the ears. They were generally characterised as vivid, clearly articulated, frequent and intrusive. In contrast, voices heard by people experiencing dissociation because of previous traumatic experiences were called pseudo-hallucinations (Brewin & Patel, 2010; McCarthy-Jones & Longden, 2015). These were internal voices but more like thoughts than voices. However, recent evidence suggests that hallucinations experienced by people diagnosed with schizophrenia and those with post-traumatic stress disorder are indistinguishable (McCarthy-Jones & Longden, 2015). The eminent writer on the history of psychiatric symptoms, German Berrios (1996), has also argued that past distinctions between true hallucinations and pseudo-hallucinations were based on poor logic.

Another rule of thumb I was taught was that certain kinds of hallucinations were much more likely to indicate a psychotic illness, particularly schizophrenia. These included: commands, such as voices telling the person to harm themselves or someone else; voices providing a running commentary about the actions of the person hearing them; and two or more people talking together about the person. These features were identified by a German psychiatrist, Kurt Schneider (1959), as so characteristic of schizophrenia that they became known as 'first-rank symptoms'. Before 2013, in both ICD and DSM diagnostic systems, the presence of one first-rank symptom was sufficient to satisfy part of the criteria for a diagnosis of schizophrenia. However, as recent evidence has suggested this conclusion wrongly identified some people as having schizophrenia, first-rank symptoms were not included in the DSM-5 (Soares-Weiser et al., 2015).

These concepts and developments are based on two centuries of European psychiatric theory and debate. Our next entranceway gives us a glimpse of this history.

Historical Views of Voices and Visions in Psychiatry

As noted in Chapter 3, in European thinking the pendulum has frequently swung backwards and forwards between spiritual versus medical or pathological explanations for voices and visions (McCarthy-Jones, 2012). From the 1600s, voice hearers in Britain challenged the authority of the Anglican church by claiming they were receiving divine guidance. Church leaders supported contemporary medical explanations for such experiences, discrediting voice hearers as being ill rather than guided by God. Meanwhile, philosophers such as John Locke (1632–1704) argued that all perceptual experiences, including religious ones, had a rational explanation (Berrios, 1996).

By the early 1800s, psychiatry began to emerge as a discipline within medicine. In 1817, French physician Jean-Étienne Dominique Esquirol used the term 'hallucination' to refer to any voice, vision or perceptual experience in another sensory modality 'for which there is no external object' (Berrios, 1996). This is almost identical to the current definition in the DSM-5, 'perception-like experiences ... without an external object'. Esquirol specifically distinguished hallucinations from illusions or delusions which had previously been lumped together. Over the following decades extended debate took place between French psychiatrists, philosophers, and theologians about whether hallucinations were inherently a sign of a biological brain problem. Although some physicians argued that Joan of Arc and St Teresa ought not to be condemned as insane, they were in a minority (Berrios, 1996). Meanwhile, in Britain, by the 1860s – the same decade that Te Kooti was incarcerated in the Chatham Islands (see Chapter 2) – psychiatrists such as Henry Maudsley stated that all hallucinations were pathological symptoms indicating mental disorder with the exception of hallucinations that occurred just before falling asleep or after waking up (Leudar & Thomas, 2000; McCarthy-Jones, 2012).

Wiremu talks about the harm caused when mental health clinicians mistakenly identify spiritual experiences as psychotic hallucinations. This harm has included denying Māori values and identity and involuntarily detaining Māori under the Mental Health Act. What about the harm caused when psychiatrists have misused definitions of hallucinations, or the potential for abuse of power when people have been involuntarily detained under mental health laws?

One example from England in the late 1800s concerns Georgina Weldon (1837–1914), a singer and supporter of women's suffrage (Owen, 1989). Georgina was a strong believer in spiritualism[1] and viewed the voices she heard as spiritual experiences. She was separated from her husband, Henry Weldon, who objected to paying maintenance. In 1878, he attempted to persuade two psychiatrists to certify Georgina as insane based solely on her previous descriptions of voice-hearing. Henry arranged to have her incarcerated in a private psychiatric hospital owned by one of the psychiatrists, for a sum of half of what he was paying in maintenance. Georgina, however, gave her would-be captors the slip and sought counsel of a magistrate who certified that she was of sound mind. One of the psychiatrists, Forbes Winslow (1844–1913), published his assessment of her case in the *British Medical Journal* in 1879, justifying his conclusion that she was insane based solely on her historical report of having heard a 'miraculous voice' and having been persuaded to act on it. In 1882, a new English law, the Married Women's Property Act, gave her legal recourse. Georgina familiarised herself with the law, represented herself in court and successfully sued Forbes Winslow. She went on to sue two other doctors who had signed her lunacy order and was awarded damages in each case (Owen, 1989).

While Georgina's story is more about unethical and abusive practice than the significance of hallucinations in mental disorder, it illustrates the importance of safeguards to protect human rights and facilitate scrutiny of ethical standards in psychiatric care.

It may be obvious to readers that women's perspectives were neither sought nor included in debates about the meaning of hallucinations in psychiatry at this time. Nor were people with lived experience of voices and visions asked to contribute. It goes without saying that Indigenous peoples, whose lives were being impacted by European colonial practices around the globe, were not consulted.

Wiremu

I don't have a problem with European philosophers trying to separate their thinking from that of the church. However, I would question their certainty about their own beliefs. They were not taking any Indigenous views into account. Māori Marsden[2] has said that the colonisation of Indigenous peoples has usually involved pacifying communities with a treaty, forcing compliance using weapons and laws, stealing land and natural resources and then using processes of assimilation to finally kill off the culture (Royal, 2003). How can we make sense of such similar approaches all over the planet? Tina Ngata (2019), a Ngāti Porou advocate for Indigenous and human rights, has pointed out that these practices can be traced back to the 1400s and a series of papal 'bulls' or laws from the Catholic Church known as the Doctrine of Discovery. These laws stated that European monarchs and their representatives could invade and conquer any foreign lands that were not under Christian control and convert or kill the inhabitants. In order to be civilised, you had to be Christianised; unless you believed in the Bible, you weren't civil. Even if you were converted, you had to disavow your culture – you had to lay it down and take up the cross. It happened to millions of people.

So how is this related to voices and visions in psychiatry? Well, European psychiatrists and philosophers who were debating whether voices and visions were only a brain problem were not consulting Indigenous peoples. There was no acknowledgement that there might be many different worldviews. European beliefs were superior and Indigenous ideas were silenced. By the time the first doctors with mental health expertise arrived in New Zealand, there was already a strong European tradition that voices and visions represented a brain problem: spirituality was disregarded, and Māori perspectives were sidelined. Psychiatry was part of the colonising culture.

Georgina Weldon's story is an example of corrupt practice. I like her style in delivering a coup de grâce against those who tried to detain her. However, I'm sure many other women were affected without being able to defend themselves. Alongside this, Māori descriptions of voices and visions were often used to justify incarcerating people, without any consideration of whether they were having wairua (spiritual) experiences.

Allister

Emil Kraepelin, Eugen Bleuler and William James

Emil Kraepelin (1856–1926) and Eugen Bleuler (1857–1939) were German psychiatrists who compiled detailed accounts of their patients' descriptions of voice hearing, visions and other experiences in the late 1800s and early 1900s (Kraepelin, 1919; Bleuler, 1950).

Kraepelin reported that hallucinations were often present when people were unwell, and 'hallucinations of hearing' were much more frequent than those of vision (Kraepelin, 1919). In the early stages of a psychotic illness, people might hear simple noises, 'rustling, buzzing, ringing in the ears', and later these would evolve into distinct and disturbing 'voices'. Some voice hearers referred to these voices as 'in the ear' or 'in the head' or sometimes elsewhere in the body, such as the belly. However, most were clear that they originated from the environment around them. Often voices would appear as sense perceptions, as if they had heard them with their ears. Other times they appeared as 'voices of conscience', or 'an inward voice in the thoughts'. Kraepelin identified that what the voices said was almost always 'unpleasant and disturbing', with teasing, mocking or abusive language, often accompanied by violent threats and commands. Some voices would comment on the thoughts and actions of the person while other voices were incomprehensible.

Kraepelin recorded the vivid language used by some of his patients. For example, one person recalled, 'the voices rushed in on me at all times like burning lions' (Kraepelin, 1919).

Unfortunately, because Kraepelin and Bleuler report only fragments of a large number of people's experiences without detailed case histories, there is no context for any particular person's experience. For people who had recounted hearing abusive voices, there is no way of knowing whether they may have experienced violence and emotional abuse in their earlier lives, and therefore whether trauma may have been a contributing factor in their illness. For those who described hearing 'voices of spirits which are quite near', or hearing 'voices of dead people' or having an 'inner feeling in the soul' (Kraepelin, 1919), it is impossible to know whether there was a meaningful context to the implication that their voices were spiritual in origin, such as having had spiritual experiences earlier in life. The implicit assumption is that almost all hallucinations were a sign of pathology, either psychiatric or neurological.

Writers such as Maudsley, Kraepelin and Bleuler dismissed any suggestion of a spiritual origin for voices and visions as they were working to strengthen the credibility of the science of psychiatry against a background of a strong popular interest in spiritualism. In contrast, systematic research of paranormal phenomena was being carried out at that time in France and Britain. These researchers were convinced that not all experiences of voices and visions were pathological. For example, in 1894 the Society for Psychical Research in the United Kingdom published a study entitled *Census of Hallucinations*. This survey of 17,000 members of the general public asked about a range of experiences, with 2.9% of respondents reporting hearing voices that others couldn't hear (Sidgwick et al., 1894). Such results were dismissed as unscientific by mainstream psychiatry.

There were other dissenters to the secular view of psychiatric theory and practice. William James (1842–1910), an American doctor, psychologist and philosopher, became critical of the 'medical materialist' thinking of his time that, in his words, 'snuffs out' St Teresa as being 'an hysteric', dismisses St Francis as 'an hereditary degenerate' and 'finishes up' St Paul by suggesting his vision on the road to Damascus was most likely 'a discharging lesion of the occipital cortex, he being an epileptic' (James, 2002).

Rejecting 'simpleminded' medical explanations for all mystical experiences, James suggested that voices or visions should be considered pathological only when they were distressing or undermining. He advocated for an examination of their 'fruits for life' (James, 2002). For example, he pointed out that St Teresa's spiritual experiences had given her more energy and tranquillity.

William James' view on 'fruits for life' reminded me of Wiremu's focus on fruits in Chapter 1, and his reaction to the experiences of the Children of Fátima in Chapter 3.

Wiremu

By the time of Emil Kraepelin, it seems to me that psychiatrists had dismissed the spiritual side as unscientific. There was no space given to allow exploration of this area. It appears that Kraepelin was determined to stay in his lane and stick to his clinical point of view. He might have heard of ghosts and spooks, but in his clinical writing didn't examine spirituality in any depth. If I had the opportunity to meet with Professor Kraepelin, I would have been curious to see if he was open to kōrero (talk) about voices and visions. Would he have listened to me if I shed a different light on them? If we met together with one of his patients who described 'voices of spirits which are quite near', would he have been open to me exploring their experiences in more detail to help understand if they were spiritual? If I could perceive what they were experiencing, a shared experience like that could convince me that they were having spiritual experiences.

I like William James' kōrero about spiritual experiences being evident when they enhance a person's life. As I said in Chapter 2, 'mā te hua ka kitea', by the fruits we can see more clearly. I tend to evaluate a person's experience based on the changes that are apparent in their life and behaviour. James goes on to talk about negative voices and visions indicating pathology. This is interesting because I'm not sure what kind of pathology he is referring to. If he means medical pathology, then I would question that. I accept that there are some medical conditions that can cause distressing voices and visions, but just because a person hears voices that bother them or sees visions that disturb them, that doesn't prove they are not having spiritual experiences.

Allister

Psychiatric Views on the Causes of Hallucinations

There have been many different conceptualisations in psychiatry about what causes hallucinations. In the 19th century, Esquirol and Maudsley suggested they might represent a disturbance of memory and imagination leading to thoughts being experienced as sensations. Meanwhile, an Italian psychiatrist, Auguste Tamburini, maintained that hallucinations were caused by irritation of specific areas of the brain cortex (Berrios, 1990). As a result, psychiatrists and neuroscientists became more focused on specific brain anatomy. Later, when it became possible to stimulate particular parts of the brain during neurosurgical procedures while the patient was still awake, it appeared that localised areas might be critical. For example, Penfield and Perot (1963) found that electrical stimulation resulted in auditory hallucinations only when they touched an electrode on the top edge of the temporal lobes, known as the superior temporal gyrus (McCarthy-Jones, 2012). Some of their patients heard buzzing or banging, some heard familiar voices, and some heard sounds of music. This depended on which part of the brain was being stimulated.

As neuroscientific observations became more sophisticated, it was suggested that certain pathways might be involved in hallucinations. For example, recent research using functional magnetic resonance imaging (fMRI) brain scans on people with auditory hallucinations has shown increased brain activity in pathways associated with speech and language processing (McCarthy-Jones, 2012).

As understanding grew about the role of chemical messengers between brain cells, it seemed that dopamine might be important because drugs that block dopamine and particular subtypes of dopamine appeared to help stop hallucinations. Recreational drugs such as cocaine and amphetamines increase dopamine levels and cause hallucinations and other symptoms such as delusions, which are hard to distinguish from a severe illness such as schizophrenia (Stahl, 2013). In addition, some drugs for treating Parkinson's stimulate dopamine pathways and tend to cause hallucinations.

More recently, psychiatrists have been interested in the role of dopamine in assigning importance or 'salience' to events and experiences, so that we can make sense of our daily lives (Kapur, 2003). According to this theory, if the levels of dopamine are increased, as occurs in schizophrenia, the salience assigned to otherwise unremarkable events becomes distorted. This means that the importance of some sensory experiences, particularly involving sight and sound, may get exaggerated, resulting in auditory and/or visual hallucinations. Meanwhile efforts by the brain to make sense of these experiences can result in delusions. Antipsychotic medication partially blocks the effects of excess dopamine, which would reduce the abnormal salience of these experiences and allow more flexible thinking and hopefully some psychological resolution.

A number of psychological theories suggest hallucinations may originate from inner speech or vivid imagery. Lev Vygotsky (1896–1934), a Russian psychologist, suggested that inner speech developed from a child learning to internalise phrases used by others in their environment (Oyebode, 2018). Cognitive researchers hypothesise that hallucinations may be fragments of inner speech which appear alien. Another theory is that hallucinations may originate from vivid imagery in people who are having difficulty recognising that their experiences are self-generated (McCarthy-Jones, 2012).

Different theories focus on memory function. For example, people may have hallucinations when memories that have been out of conscious awareness are unexpectedly activated and then perceived to come from outside the person. This is particularly relevant to understanding the link between traumatic experiences and hallucinations. According to one theory, memories of events are initially encoded in short-term memory and then processed by our brains, allowing them to be integrated into our sense of ourselves and the world. When the memory is distressing, disturbing emotions, images, thoughts and body sensations can interfere with our brain's ability to integrate these memories (Shapiro, 2001). Traumatic memories can then become stuck in a raw unprocessed form and easily triggered by reminders of the event, resulting in intrusive recollections such as flashbacks and nightmares. This theory could explain hallucinations which resemble fragments of auditory or visual memories. Flashbacks occur while the person is awake and may include such fragments. They are often vivid, with a compelling sense of reality, as if they were happening at that moment. They may feel very frightening and threatening. However, most people with post-traumatic stress disorder (PTSD) who hear voices don't hear or see fragments of actual memories (McCarthy-Jones & Longden, 2015).

Another theory focused on people who experience severe and repeated traumatic experiences in childhood describes how this can lead to parts of their mind being separated off from each other (van der Hart et al., 2010). Such dissociative protection is believed to prevent the person being overwhelmed by repeatedly re-experiencing terrifying traumatic memories. Those parts of a person can appear to resemble human personality characteristics. For example, if one part is perceiving the angry or critical expression of another part as a hostile voice or vision, its origin could be obscured and interpreted as arising from somewhere external to the person.

One problem for many of these theories is that the proposed changes in brain structure and function appear to be enduring, yet hallucinations are intermittent. It seems that while neuroscience has made some significant advances, much more remains to be discovered in this field. As Wiremu has expressed in this book, all these theories are secular. Western research is generally searching for explanations of voices and visions only in the places that fit with non-spiritual paradigms.

Voices and Visions in Psychiatric and Other Medical Conditions

Every medical practitioner is likely to have met people who experienced hallucinations because they were physically unwell. These people may have been acutely confused or delirious or may have taken substances. Clinical observations like these offer compelling evidence to me as a doctor that hallucinations can be caused by biological changes in the brain. Here we look at three causes of voices and visions: psychiatric conditions, substance use and brain problems.

While hallucinations are a core symptom in schizophrenia, they are also common in other psychiatric conditions. On average, more than half of people diagnosed with schizophrenia are reported to experience auditory hallucinations when unwell and one-quarter have visual hallucinations (Waters et al., 2014). More than a quarter of people with mood disorders report hearing voices during severe episodes, with a smaller percentage of people experiencing visions. Similarly, people with severe PTSD symptoms commonly have to cope with distressing hallucinations (McCarthy-Jones & Longden, 2015).

As noted in Chapter 1, substances can cause people to hear voices and see visions while intoxicated and during withdrawal states. For example, alcohol withdrawal after long-term use often results in visual hallucinations which may be fleeting or intense and prolonged. Sudden withdrawal of benzodiazepine medications such as diazepam or Valium can also result in a similar pattern of visual hallucinations. Hallucinogenic drugs are often taken by people because of their ability to cause transient but marked perceptual changes, and visual hallucinations are very common.

In contrast to the prominence of voices in psychotic conditions, visual hallucinations are more commonly associated with medical conditions. People with Parkinson's, for example, are twice as likely to have visual hallucinations than to hear voices and other sounds (Waters et al., 2014).

People who have had small blood vessel blockages to critical brain areas may experience complex visual hallucinations, such as seeing people they don't recognise dressed in unusual clothing (Manford & Andermann, 1998). In contrast, visual hallucinations associated with epilepsy are more often brief, similar each time and made up of fragments rather than whole visual images. Brain trace recordings suggest that these seizures originate in brain areas responsible for interpreting visual stimuli (Manford & Andermann, 1998). When people report hearing voices as part of a seizure, the origin is almost always seizure activity in the temporal lobes, an area of the brain responsible for making sense of sounds. People who experience voices due to a medical condition of their brain are much less likely to report voices that focus on their moral or emotional dilemmas (Braun et al., 2003).

Voices and Visions Which Are Not Considered to Indicate a Psychiatric or Medical Problem

In the general community, more than 5 percent of people report experiencing visual hallucinations (Waters et al., 2014). Surveys of auditory verbal hallucinations suggest that up to 3 percent of people report hearing voices, and two-thirds of these people do not report impairment in relation to their experiences (Sidgwick et al., 1894; Tien, 1991; McCarthy-Jones, 2012). Without impairment, by definition, they would not meet criteria for a psychiatric disorder. As discussed above, it is helpful to be aware of voices and visions that are not a sign of a problem and to understand what these experiences can be like. Voices during sleep onset can include hearing your name, brief friendly or unfriendly comments from a strange or familiar voice, or nonsensical statements (McCarthy-Jones, 2012). Visions while waking up are common and may consist of spots of light or geometric shapes or more complex images such as animals and human figures. People having these experiences may feel curious, neutral or afraid (Manford & Andermann, 1998).

Voices or visions experienced shortly after the death of a loved one are also not considered pathological in psychiatry. It is common for older adults to see a partner who has died shortly after their death (Elsaesser et al., 2021). In the psychiatric literature, these experiences are commonly assumed to be visual hallucinations (Sadock & Sadock, 2005).

In surveys of doctors and nurses working with dying people in the United States and India, a significant number reported having worked with people close to death who appeared to, or said they had seen, people others couldn't see (Osis & Haraldsson, 1977). The majority of those described seeing deceased relatives, others they knew, or a religious figure that was important to them.

Wiremu

When psychiatrists talk about normal hallucinations just before and after sleep, I have a different interpretation. I believe we are more open to wairua experiences at those times. My view is that just before going to sleep, a spiritual doorway can open up, and people may then see and hear things spiritually that wouldn't be otherwise apparent to them.

When a person's spouse dies, it is natural that they may want to see their loved one again. Perhaps seeing their deceased partner could be due to that yearning resulting in them imagining it. However, there is another possibility. It is fairly common for our loved ones to appear to us just after they have passed away. That's wairua. It's not just spouses. I have seen people shortly after their deaths, often within an hour of their passing. The first time I had that experience was when I was 12 and living in Tiniroto. One night I was walking up to visit a mate whose Dad owned the local tavern. In the darkness I could see a figure walking past me and recognised him as a local man who drove a truck in our area. There was something different about his movement and appearance that made me feel scared. When I got to the pub, people were talking about this man and how he had driven his truck off the road and died at the scene of the accident. This experience had nothing to do with yearning or a close relationship. I didn't even like the man.

With regards to people seeing visions on their deathbed, I would think it is very common. Scientists have hypothesised that this might be due to the brain having a mechanism to ease the psychological pain of the dying process. The idea is that the brain creates an illusion that everything is okay, and your family is waiting there. However, I believe that when it's time for you to die, your people will come back for you. I gave an example of this in Chapter 2, when I spoke about 'ā wairua' and the ancestors I sensed there at the time that my sister Pare died.

Allister

Cultural and Spiritual Interpretations of Hallucinations

If Wiremu is right, and there are people in our communities who have spiritual experiences that relate to the presence of their ancestors or other spirits, what research findings can help guide psychiatrists and other mental health clinicians in their practice? Some relevant research comes from the field of anthropology.

Tanya Luhrmann, an American anthropologist, has studied voices and visions in a range of cultural settings. Following research with charismatic Christians in the United States, she collaborated with researchers in Ghana and India to examine how people with a diagnosis of schizophrenia (based on DSM criteria) in these three diverse settings described their voices (Luhrmann, 2012; Luhrmann et al., 2015; Larøi et al., 2014). Voice hearers in the United States were more tormented by their voices and viewed them as evidence that they were 'crazy'. Voice hearers in India were less likely to view their voices as 'bad' even when they disliked them. Some assumed their voices were relations who might be, for example instructing them to do housework. Those in Ghana commonly identified their main voice as 'God'. These voices were often viewed as positive, and some advised them to ignore bad or mean voices. These strikingly divergent interpretations of hallucinations by people from these cultural settings raise many questions about the impact of different interpretations of voices and visions on people's wellbeing. It is worth noting that previous multi-site World Health Organisation research found that people with a diagnosis of schizophrenia in Africa or India had better clinical and social outcomes than those in Europe or North America (Leff et al., 1992).

Elsewhere, Tanya Luhrmann and different colleagues have distinguished three patterns of hearing voices (Larøi et al., 2014; Luhrmann, 2017). The first pattern was found in voice hearers from religious groups who reported hearing the voice of God. They described hearing short, guiding or affirming statements on rare occasions only. They may have felt surprised, even startled, but not harassed. The second pattern was in people with a diagnosis of schizophrenia who heard voices frequently, often many times an hour, and found them highly distressing. The third group were religious experts who had equally intense and frequent voices as the second group, but without distress or other symptoms of psychosis.

Wiremu

When Tanya Luhrmann refers to a group of people with many distressing voices and visions, my first response is that some of those people may be having spiritual experiences. Even though they may feel negative, to me it's possible the person may find meaning in them, even years down the track. The religious experts that Tanya Luhrmann talks about in her third group appear to have found a way to put their spiritual experiences to use. My view is that if the person doesn't have a way of making sense of such experiences and can't put them to proper use, they may experience a state of confusion and fear. I will outline my approach to understanding such situations in Chapter 9.

Allister

Differentiating Spiritual Experiences from Psychosis

Recent studies have started to provide evidence that could be used in a clinical interview to help people figure out if they are having spiritual experiences or have a mental health problem.

Moseley et al. (2022) compared the voice-hearing experiences of people with psychosis with people from spiritualist communities in Britain. Most participants in the spiritual group were white women. The researchers found that the spiritual group began hearing voices at a younger age than the psychosis group, often in early childhood. The spiritual group described experiences in other sensory modalities at the same time as hearing voices;

for instance, seeing something or having a tactile feeling believed to be from the same entity causing the voices. Such reports were much less common in the psychosis group. The spiritual group was more likely to report being aware of a 'felt presence'.

People in the spiritual group described seeing visual imagery with their 'mind's eye', which they associated with their voices. This was very uncommon in the psychosis group. Although both groups experienced voices which were externally located, the psychosis group was much more likely than the spiritual group to report voices coming through doors or walls.

There was a marked difference between the groups in their sense of agency in relation to their voices. Over the years, members of the spiritual group were able to exert influence over their voices by tuning in and engaging them in dialogue. This group was much more likely than the psychosis group to feel that their voices' content was positive and to feel positive emotions about this content. Alongside this, a number of the spiritual group said that the onset of their voices had been during a difficult time, such as parental separation or bereavement.

Further research has investigated childhood experiences in people who in their adult life identified as spiritualist mediums. One study focused on in-depth interviews with ten spiritualist mediums and found that nine of the participants reported experiences such as voice hearing, visions, and seeing auras from a young age (Roxburgh & Roe, 2014). These experiences included reports of seeing 'spirit children', other people, and 'apparitions of animals'. A number grew up in environments where such experiences were normalised, for example, by family members or acquaintances. For many the onset of their voices and visions occurred at a challenging time in their life and initially they found it disturbing.

Over time, participants recalled finding ways to live with and regulate their experiences. Some described spirits guiding them: for example, mentoring them to manage negative spirit voices that might otherwise be troubling. One participant used the metaphor of an open book to describe her method of controlling the influence of spirits in her life, saying that when she was not working as a medium, it was important for her to 'close the book' to protect her wellbeing. Another used a similar metaphor to Wiremu's kūaha or doorway, stating, 'The door is ajar. I know I've pulled it closed, but it's unlocked so if they [spirit voices] need to come through they can sort of knock on that door and push it open and say, "We're here"' (Roxburgh & Roe, 2014).

Wiremu

I'm interested in the findings of the research comparing people with spiritual experiences with those labelled as having psychosis. The point about visual imagery captures my attention. Experienced matekite (those with spiritual awareness) can develop their visual imagery as a tool. Sometimes I get a visual image that comes to mind, and I realise that it relates to someone I'm yet to meet in my healing mahi. That's a skill in my kete (basket) that sits there till I need it. I may see that in the wairua several days beforehand. That image may tell me something about the person nobody else knows, even those who are closest to them. When I raise that with them, the result may be a feeling of hope or faith which can lift them on their healing journey.

With a visual perception, I may see something – for example, someone's ancestor – as if they were located in space beside the person. In contrast, when I feel a presence, I can become aware of an entity present in space without necessarily seeing, hearing or touching it. I know it's there. I can describe its location in the room, even behind me. It's like a kind of intuitive radar. This allows me to home in on it, to see what else I can perceive. As I focus on it, I adjust my senses to the room, the ambient lighting, sounds and warmth. I may then pick up a fuzzy visual perception, and if I sit with it more details become clear.

Voice hearers labelled with psychosis often seem to hear harsh voices, abusive voices, berating them. They don't tell them they are beautiful or loved. I don't generally hear negative voices. A high percentage of the voices I hear are positive and relate to my tīpuna (ancestors). I usually hear voices in my immediate vicinity. I can't recall hearing any voices coming through a wall or door. Sometimes I may hear them coming from far off in the distance. For example, I sometimes hear distant voices that relate to a particular person, perhaps two or three days before meeting them.

In the spiritual group, their first experiences were at an early age. I often hear matekite or people with spiritual awareness say that they first heard or saw things when they were little. When I was young, I had many imaginary friends. Sometimes they would be there sitting on the branches of trees. We call them patupaiarehe (fairy folk). My kuia also knew they were there and reassured me.

I believe it is often the case that matekite experiences can begin due to some difficulties or trauma. For me, being a whāngai (extended family adoptee) was a traumatic loss, even as a pēpē (baby). Even though I was well looked after by my mother, Nancy, and my kuia, for years I felt that I had been given away because I was unwanted, and I wonder if that contributed to my early wairua experiences.

Allister

Bringing Spirituality into Mental Health Care

For those of us working in psychiatry and mental health, is there intellectual and emotional space for us to engage with the spiritual experiences and religious values of the people we work with? In the past some psychiatrists have believed they should avoid conversations about religion and spirituality, perhaps to protect patients from doctors proselytising their own religious views (Poole et al., 2019). In cultures with individualistic values, such as the dominant European and American cultures, it may be considered intrusive to inquire about someone's personal religious views. From these points of view, offering to start a psychiatric interview with a culturally appropriate prayer or other spiritual opening may be considered inappropriate and perhaps a violation of professional boundaries.

As Wiremu has pointed out, secular thinking and approaches in psychiatry have contributed to Indigenous values being rendered invisible. Secular mental health environments may feel hostile and alien for Indigenous peoples (Durie, 1998; Tamasese et al., 2005). In Aotearoa, Māori health leaders have advocated for greater consideration of Māori worldviews, experiences and approaches in mental health care. These include people with lived experience of mental distress, tohunga, academics, psychologists and psychiatrists (Bidois, 2017; Durie, 1998, 2011; Huirama, 2019; Kingi et al., 2017; Ngata, 2014; Rangihuna et al., 2018; Royal, 2003; Waitoki & Levy, 2016).

Psychiatrists globally have been vocal in advocating for a more sophisticated approach to considering spirituality and religion in psychiatry and mental health assessment and treatment (Cook et al., 2009; Cook, 2013; Thatikonda, 2019). As a result, the World Psychiatric Association (WPA) published a position statement on religion and spirituality in psychiatry noting that religion and spirituality are relevant for the majority of the world's population, and most people wish for their spiritual values to be taken into account in their health care (Moreira-Almeida et al., 2016). The statement calls for psychiatrists to tactfully consider people's religious and spiritual values in history-taking. It asserts that understanding the significance of religion and spirituality for psychiatric diagnosis, aetiology and treatment should be 'essential components in psychiatric training and professional development'. It also calls for research into the impact of religions and spirituality on psychiatry covering a 'wide diversity of cultural and geographical' settings. My interpretation of the WPA position statement's relevance for Aotearoa is that it advocates for bringing an understanding of Māori spirituality to all aspects of mental health care for Māori individuals and whānau. Furthermore, it is suggesting that spirituality may be important for many people as part of their mental health care, regardless of their cultural background.

Conclusion

We have entered a number of doorways in Western psychiatry to look at the meaning of voices and visions. We have seen that European psychiatric interpretations of voices and visions as hallucinations were consolidated by the mid-to-late 1800s. As Wiremu explained, these theories have been exported to other parts of the world and have become part of the colonial legacy of psychiatry. Spiritual meanings had already been excluded as unscientific, resulting in a deep divide between accepted knowledge in psychiatry and Māori and other Indigenous understandings. Doctors and psychiatrists have been persuaded by evidence that voices and visions can arise from organic brain problems and psychosis. In psychiatry and psychology, theories about the origin of hallucinations have focused on brain pathways, neurotransmitter theories, and hypotheses about inner speech, vivid imagery, memory and trauma.

So how can this divide be addressed? If in psychiatry we have no knowledge about spiritual voices and visions, and a significant proportion of people who hear voices could be hearing spiritual voices or seeing spiritual visions – is our lack of knowledge and awareness a problem?

I (Allister) think it is. Many readers may have better ideas for ways to address this divide. Two obvious pathways occur to me. One is for psychiatrists and other mental health clinicians to develop the practice of working in partnership with Māori practitioners with wairua expertise, or with non-Māori spiritual practitioners, so that we can offer more informed assessments and interventions for people who come to us with distressing voices and visions. The second is for Māori-led research to be supported to explore what happens for people who see visions and hear voices and look at how these experiences are related to wairua.

In the next chapter, Egan's account of his early life experiences of wairua and then his treatment as a young man for severe mental distress raises many questions for me as a psychiatrist about the intersection between wairua, psychosis, trauma, healing and psychiatry.

Notes

1 Spiritualists in Britain generally believe that it is possible to perceive and receive communication from people after death and that such experiences can be nurtured and developed (Moseley et al., 2022).

2 Māori Marsden (1924–1993) was a tohunga, philosopher and Anglican minister from the Tai Tokerau peoples in the far north of Aotearoa.

5 Egan

Egan Bidois, Wiremu NiaNia, and Allister Bush

Wiremu

Ahakoa te teitei o rākau	Although the tree is tall and majestic
ki te topea ka hinga	When it is cut it will fall.
Ahakoa te teitei o maunga	Even though the mountain is lofty and imposing
Ka taea e tangata te eke	Determination will carry someone to the summit
Ahakoa herea te matekite e te ture	Yet a matekite (seer) may be bound by the system
Kāore e hinga ka tū	And they shall not fall but will stand
Ka manawaroa ka ora	They will persevere and thrive
Toitū te mana	Let your mana (spiritual authority) stand
Toitū te mauri	Let your mauri (life force) stand
Haumi ē! Hui ē!	
Taiki ē!	

Allister

Egan Bidois was a colleague at Te Whare Mārie for five years, working in our Māori child adolescent and family service (CAFS) team as a community liaison worker and then taking on a kairangahau or research position at our service. I noticed he was knowledgeable about te ao Māori (the Māori world) and would speak out in our multi-disciplinary team meetings if he thought we needed to consider matters pertaining to wairua (spirit). While Wiremu tended to remain silent about such matters in the early days that I knew him, Egan was vocal and passionate in his advocacy.

Egan would accompany Wiremu on consultations and house blessings, and I could tell he had great respect for Wiremu's perspectives on the wellbeing of those they were meeting. Wiremu's humble and low-key approach often confused me. When I gradually became aware of the spiritual healing methods he was using and started to see some very positive results, I became curious. One day I had an opportunity to observe the

DOI: 10.4324/9781003187042-5

work of a tohunga (Māori healer) who worked near Te Whare Mārie. It struck me that there were strong similarities between her healing work and Wiremu's practice. However, when I asked Wiremu outright if he was a tohunga, he brushed my question aside by saying that label was reserved for special people. Finally, I had a conversation with Egan about this. When I asked him about Wiremu and my question, his response was, 'Yes, he is a tohunga. We have a saying, "Kāore te kūmara e kōrero mō tōna ake reka", which means "the kūmara does not speak of its own sweetness."'

It has been a privilege for me to learn about Egan's life and experiences in the writing of this chapter. During all our time working together, I never heard him talking about the stories he shares here. First, Egan describes his early life, his experiences of wairua during his childhood and the guidance he was given by his mother and others. He goes on to relay the circumstances of his move to university in a big city, then his situation as a student when he first became unwell. He then recounts the treatment and abusive experiences he had in a psychiatric hospital.

Reading Egan's narrative could well be distressing for some readers, especially for those who have their own lived experience of trauma and/or mental health problems and treatment. Please take care of yourself in whatever ways you find appropriate.

After Egan tells his story and shares his perspectives, Wiremu and I reflect on this moving narrative, and Egan offers his closing words.

Egan

Early Life

Egan is a Celtic name.[1] Apparently, it means fiery or ardent one. It is probably appropriate. Sometimes you can be cursed by a name. The name Bidois is from a French whaler who married into the tribe many years ago. Chances are any Bidois you bump into in New Zealand will be Māori.

I am the youngest of four living siblings. I have two older brothers and a sister. Prior to me being born I had a second sister, but she passed away early in her life. She ended up drowning in a local river. Even though I did not know her physically, this sister is one of the constant voices that I hear. She is a kaitiaki, a guardian, and is with me all the time. A couple of people have asked me, 'How do you know it is your sister's voice if you have never heard her voice?' I just know it is.

My nana, my kuia (grandmother) on my Dad's side, lived in Te Puna in the Bay of Plenty. We would often drive up to visit her for holidays. She passed away when I was nine or ten. I think it was about a month after her passing that she popped in for the first time and spoke to me. She has been present with me ever since. My kuia is another one of my constant voices.

My mother has similar experiences to those I've had all my life. She can sense things around her. She is certainly a very spiritual person. I find this interesting given her vocation as a psychiatric nurse. I sometimes wondered if she had some internal conflict given that she was trained to view things in a medical way. My mum was my main support growing up because I knew she could understand what I was experiencing. When I was a baby, other people would be carrying me around and I would be looking over their shoulder and cooing at something in the corner. They would comment on it, perhaps wondering what I was doing. My mum would tell them, 'It's okay. He is just seeing stuff'. In my late 20s, I asked my mother about those times and whether she ever told people what I was seeing. She replied that she never did as these experiences were for me personally and not them. In addition, she didn't expect they would understand it.

My mother was active within various spiritual groups where we lived in Tūrangi, at the southern end of Lake Taupō, in the North Island. Quite often she would go with a rōpū (group) to visit a house that needed blessing and would take me along as well. My role was to be a spotter. They would send me into the house with the elders. For me it was like a game. I would see something in a room, and I would yell out, 'Koro, it's in here!' And then, 'Oh no, it's moving!' And I would chase it. I can still recall some of the things I would see. For example, I remember seeing a person, fully dressed, so clear to me that they looked like a real flesh-and-blood person. Or else I might see an older lady with white hair and brown eyes, sitting in a lounge chair and holding her walking stick. It was very specific. Other times I might not get such a clear visual impression.

My earliest memory of seeing something was from when I was three. I saw a tall, golden pillar of light standing at the foot of my bed. Even though I could not see any facial features or anything like that, it felt male. It felt to me like it was facing towards me and watching over me. I remember telling my Mum that there was this golden man standing at the end of my bed. Her response was, 'That's okay. They are called apa (angels).'

Perhaps two months later, I recall waking and seeing a second pillar of light, this time standing off to one side. This apa felt female to me. The male one was also there. This time my experience was quite different. Both of them were facing away from me towards my bedroom window. At that moment I had a most foreboding and chilling feeling. I could sense something coming from outside of the house. The only word I have to explain that feeling I had was that it was evil. I could sense that whatever that thing was, it was now directly outside my bedroom window. The next thing I recall was seeing these two golden pillars of light merging together. A moment later they formed this great big ball of golden light and roared out the window and, in a flash, the evil thing was gone. As I think back on this experience so many years later, the only thing I can surmise is that these two beings were waiting and keeping an eye on me until this thing showed up, in order to protect me. And when it did turn up, they took it out.

It was when I started school that I first remember feeling different from others. I recall one day playing with other kids in the playground and asking a boy, 'Hey, who is this old lady with you?' Looking taken aback, he replied, 'What old lady?' I responded, 'The old lady standing behind you.' But he couldn't see her and looked confused.

People thought I was a freak. By the age of seven I had only a very small group of friends. I remember one day that year coming to school, and I noticed a girl in our class. I immediately sensed something was wrong for her. Not only that; I could feel her emitting pain. Then when I focused on her I saw what had been done to her the previous night. She'd been sexually molested. I could absolutely feel it, and I could see that occurring. At morning break I bowled up to her and gave her a hug. She looked surprised and asked me why I hugged her. I replied, 'That was for what was done to you last night. I am really sorry about what happened.' At that point she totally freaked out. When I look back now, I can see that her reaction was absolutely understandable. Growing up, when you can see and hear things about the private lives of others like this, you've got to learn wisdom about what you share and what you do not. She did not need to hear me say that.

My parents never mentioned these sorts of experiences to our family doctor. We only ever consulted them about physical health problems. Fortunately, I was never subjected to any medical or psychiatric assessment. It was just seen as who I was within my family. Having said that, I also recall moments in which I felt shunned by the extended whānau (family). I remember being at one of our marae (Māori meeting houses) for a tangi (bereavement ritual). Some of the younger kids were teasing me. A koroua (male elder) reprimanded them, 'Hey don't pick on him, leave him alone!' At first, I thought, how awesome; this koro (male elder) is standing up for me. However, the next thing he said troubled me for a long time. He said, 'Don't do that because he will curse you.' Those kids grew up with this fear of me having some sort of ability to curse them, as if I was some kind of witch doctor. I felt quite ostracised within my culture at that time.

These days my usual experiences are that I hear three voices. Off to the left of me is my sister, Bobby. Off to the right of me is my nanny. Then there is a new one which just joined: someone who passed away recently. I am very happy this person is with me. What do I see? A friend of mine asked me this question once. He enquired, 'Can you describe to me what you see and how you see things?' My response was, 'Bro, can you remember when we were growing up at school and we had those overhead projectors? It was like early PowerPoint transparencies that would project up onto a wall. My reality is that it is like I am seeing a transparency. However, I am not just seeing one sheet; I may see up to 11 sheets. And on every single one of those sheets may be a separate reality, just moving constantly in and out of focus.' My friend asked me, 'So what are those realities?' I replied, 'Well I believe that they are the past, the present, the future and alternative versions of each. Or none of that. So yeah, seeing that can be quite distracting.'

Sensory Overload

It was not until I left Hautu village in Tūrangi to study in Hamilton, a bigger city a couple of hours' drive north of Tūrangi, that things began to get really troubling. Looking back, I realise I was not ready for the amount of energy I'd be sensing. When I am around someone, while I would physically see one person, I'd see via wairua multiple other entities, energies and even events around and concerning them. I might sense if they are carrying some form of pain or trauma. Moving from a very small community with a generally manageable amount of additional input to a university community with 10,000 other people, I realise now that my senses became overloaded. I just couldn't deal with it. It got to the point when I would be walking through university and hearing voices everywhere. I would look around and I would see a person walking along but there were ten other entities with that person. And it was at that time that my visual experiences started to feel more horrific. If I focused on someone, I might see pain that had been inflicted on them, or pain they had inflicted on other people. I found these experiences very difficult to deal with.

Strangely enough, growing up in the central North Island, I'd never touched marijuana. Some people might think that is very surprising. Marijuana was considered to be the main growth industry in Tūrangi at the time. However, it wasn't long before I went to a student party when I was at university in Hamilton, and I was offered a joint. I turned it down. The following week at another party, people were smoking dope and again I was offered some. Once more I turned it down. Not long after, someone I was acquainted with offered me a joint and insisted, 'Bro, just take a puff. You need to settle down. We can see you're not relaxed.' This time I did try it.

The next morning, I was intrigued to discover that I couldn't hear any voices. I set off on a walk through the university campus and found that when I saw a person, I didn't see any other things with that person. I thought this was awesome. Maybe marijuana was what I needed!

After this realisation, I began smoking small amounts of marijuana: enough to kill off the visions, suppress the voices, prevent all those unpleasant experiences and help me sleep. The voices don't stop just because you are asleep. I found I could sleep more peacefully if I smoked a joint. Initially marijuana helped me out. However, before long the experiences came back. The voices came back louder. The things I could see came back clearer and more horrific.

I would like to think I am a reasonably intelligent man. However, at this time my logic led me astray. I concluded I just needed more marijuana. When I smoked more, the same thing happened. All the voices and visions disappeared temporarily, but eventually they returned. This time they would come back louder, faster, harder and more painful; more intense. It got to the point that it didn't matter how much I smoked. After some weeks I was smoking so much pot it would have made Cheech and Chong look like choirboys.[2]

It was then that I began to have much more disturbing experiences. For example, I remember being in a law lecture and turning to this guy and saying, 'Nah, thanks, mate; I've got one.' The man next to me looked at me puzzled and asked, 'What?' I explained, 'I've got a pen, but thank you, mate.' He just stared at me and said, 'Excuse me?' I elaborated, 'You just sat down, and you asked me if I needed a pen, because you had a spare one.' His response was, 'Bro, I just sat down. I haven't said anything to you.' I wasn't fazed at all. I just replied, 'Sweet as.'

In another lecture I became aware of a guy sitting two seats to the right of me. After some time, I started to think he was trying to mess with my head. I could hear him whispering at me, yet as soon as I looked at him, he would close his mouth. I could hear him mutter, 'Hey, look at me, look at me!' I would turn to him, and immediately his mouth was closed, and he was looking at the board. A moment later he would be at it again. I could hear him whisper, 'Hey, look at me again; look at me.' So I looked at him once more and, just as before, he had his mouth closed.

Before long, I conceived this marvellous plan. I decided that if I got to the law lectures really, really early, I could get right up to the back row and I could keep an eye on everyone. And if anyone played their whisper shut-up games, I'll be able to spot them. So that's what I did for a while. It was brilliant. No one tried to mess with my head; no one was trying to whisper and shut up when I looked at them. However, soon after I became much more stressed out with our mid-year law exam approaching.

Two weeks out from the exam, I had been studying really hard. I was feeling very stressed out and not sleeping well. Arriving early to my law lecture, I noticed three guys already seated up in the back row. A couple of rows down from them was a mate I went to school with. He waved out to me. 'Egan, come here. Sit by me.' So I moved over to the seat beside him. He asked me how I was. I replied, 'I am pretty stressed obviously' and talked about the exam coming up. Otherwise, I said I was doing okay.

Then he enquired, 'Bro, I have got to ask you a question. At Phil's party, how drunk were you?' I replied, 'I was drunk as. Cut to the gills.' He looked at me and continued, 'How stoned were you?' I responded, 'I was flying like a kite, bro.' He went on, 'I figured that because you were saying and doing some really crazy stuff. You were freaking a whole bunch of people out. They were coming up to me and saying, "What is wrong with your boy? Man! Far out!" I reassured them, "No he is just stoned, man, he's just pissed. He is a good guy."' He searched my face and asked once again, 'But you are okay, bro?' I said, 'Yeah, I was just pissed and stoned.' He nodded, 'Cool as, bro.'

Midway through this lecture the three dudes in the back row started just talking about nothing. I was trying to focus on the lecture, knowing the exam was coming up. When they kept raising their voices, I began to feel quite irritated. Finally, I turned around to shush them. I put my index finger to my lips and said, 'Shush!' No sooner had I done that when I heard one of them say, 'Did he just shush us? Does he think we are five years old? What the heck?' They kept on yakking. Before long I was quite annoyed, but I kept my cool and being all polite turned and motioned again for them to shush. I turned back around to the front and tried to focus on what the lecturer was saying. Meanwhile I heard one of them behind me say, 'He did just try to shush us. What a dick!' The other guy growled, 'Just go down there and punch him in the back of the head.' I thought 'What? These guys want to have a fight? Okay!'

I put down my pen; I stood up. I turned around slowly and raised my voice. 'You guys want to have a go at me?' I pointed at them, getting ready to take them on. Suddenly my mate was grabbing hold of me, saying, 'Bro what are you doing?' Outraged, I explained, 'Mate! These guys up the back want to have a go at me!' But he wasn't listening, telling me, 'Bro, just calm down!' I insisted, 'These dudes up the back are challenging me. They wanna step me out. They want to smash me!' My mate was staring intently at me and asked, 'What dudes?' I was adamant, 'Those dudes in the back row.' His response floored me. 'There is nobody there, bro; there is nobody there!'

First Psychiatric Admission

Not long after that day, I found myself in the accident and emergency department of the local hospital in Hamilton. I was having a chat with a really tall guy in a nice suit. Having worked in mental health now for about 20 years, I know that guy would have been a duty registrar; a trainee psychiatrist doing an assessment on me. He asked me a whole bunch of questions. The next thing I knew I was in the back of a police patrol car, taking a quick trip south of Hamilton to Tokanui Psychiatric Hospital.

I was just 18, and this was my first psychiatric admission. I was originally committed under the Mental Health Act for an assessment for drug-induced psychosis. Of course, with the amount of pot I was smoking, it was surmised that I was experiencing this psychotic break as a consequence of drugs. When the drugs were out of my system and I was still experiencing those supposed psychotic breaks, I was deemed to have paranoid schizophrenia. The reality for me was I was seeing and hearing things well before I smoked my first joint. My voices and visions didn't originate at that time. I will acknowledge that abusing that substance drove me into realms of sensory experiences that I couldn't deal with. So in some ways the system was right: it was marijuana that had created the destabilisation and psychotic break. However, I was coping relatively fine with my experiences prior to that.

During my six months in Tokanui, my psychiatrists had great difficulty finding medications that would gain control of my voices and visions. At one point, I was prescribed four different antipsychotics as well as three different sedatives. Eventually the doses were increased so much that I was at the maximum or higher than the maximum recommended daily dose for each one of them. As a result, for prolonged periods I was experiencing considerable drug toxicity. I gained almost 40 kilograms over four months. When you are on that kind and that amount of medication, you just have to *think* about food to grow another butt. It just happens.

I felt like a drug-locked zombie. I was so sedated that it required a couple of orderlies to come and collect me from my room and assist me to walk to the day room. I couldn't move. I couldn't speak. The worst part of this experience for me was that I couldn't disengage from the constant barrage of overwhelming stimuli from the voices, visions and feelings I was experiencing. It was not shutting down the voices I was hearing, and it was not shutting down my feelings. If anything, my feelings were actually amplified by the medication.

By shutting down my physical movement, the medication prevented me from using some of my main coping methods. Prior to that, and later in my life, I have often condensed and then dispersed strong sensory feelings with focused physical movement. Examples that work well for me include walking barefoot upon the grass, gardening to literally ground myself via my hands, cleansing myself by walking into the awa (river) and cupping handfuls of water over my head as I recite karakia (prayers), or isolating myself from other people and unleashing my strong feelings with fierce, focused haka[3] or taiaha practice (a Māori martial art). None of these methods were now possible.

What was I hearing? A million and one screaming voices. They were extremely derogatory voices. They were telling me, 'You are a piece of shit. Kill yourself! Die! Right now; you do not deserve life,' over and over. I was hearing the most repugnant stuff being said about other people. Someone would walk into the room. One voice would kick off and start swearing about that person. It would be calling them the most repugnant names. I was feeling things touching me and poking me and cutting through me. It was like barbed wire was running through my body.

I need to be really upfront about something here. I absolutely acknowledge that some people find hospitalisation helpful. I absolutely acknowledge that people who go to work in health services are not doing it to harm people. They're not in it for the money, so the reason they are doing it is that they have a compassionate calling. These events took place in 1990. Thankfully, within a few years of this, reforms to mental health services in New Zealand meant that horror stories that you hear coming out of places like Tokanui weren't occurring as regularly. I'm just putting that out there before I start talking in more detail about my treatment and management in Tokanui at that time.

Institutional Racism

Sometime in the mid-to-late 1990s I managed to get access to a number of my old patient files. I was motivated to do this after connecting with people who were involved with New Zealand's consumer movement. This was a group of people who had lived experience of mental distress and were working together to advocate for the rights of people using mental health services and for the improvement and transformation of these services.

I often found reading through these case notes intensely painful. I remember reading nursing notes giving their viewpoint: their summary of what my behaviours were like. The narrative of my unwellness in these patient files was constructed from a very specific lens. There were a number of examples where staff observations were certainly not congruent with my experiences at the time. For instance, one entry recorded: 'Patient was out in the yard, yelling and screaming, gesticulating wildly, yelling violent obscenities, punching at the air.' My reality was I was doing a haka. I had so much energy I could feel it coming up through the ground. It was running through my body; I could feel all this energy burning within me. I took myself out into the yard to allow it to dissipate back into the ground. I specifically chose that yard because there was nobody else there. I broke out into doing this haka, *Ka Mate*, over and over, with so much energy to try to burn it up. I was taken away to a seclusion room and locked up for three days because they viewed me as a threat.

Another entry read: 'Patient has an anal fascination. Constantly talking about anuses and bums.' I believe this comment was related to an incident in which I had no pillow. When I asked for a pillow, they brought me a cushion. My response was, 'I don't actually want a cushion. Can you get me a pillow?' They replied, 'No, you can have that cushion.' I tried to explain, 'No, I don't want to use a cushion. Our head is seen as a very sacred part. There is no way we should be laying it down on a cushion, which is where your nono, where your kumu, where your bottom sits.' I was requesting a bit more cultural appreciation. This didn't result in a seclusion event, thankfully. It did not result in me getting a pillow though.

A further entry read: 'Patient staring at the wall, muttering incomprehensible word salad and gibberish. Was asked to be quiet.' I was reciting karakia: I was saying prayers to calm myself and manage what was going on for me, to seek protection and safety within these experiences. Staring blankly at the wall was me focusing on my karakia. The incomprehensible gibberish was te reo Māori, one of the official languages of this country. Their method of asking me to be quiet was that a staff member came in, grabbed me by my long hair, pulled my head back and screamed in my face, 'Shut up, [N-word]!' That's hardly asking me to be quiet. The fact that they used the N-word suggests to me that they probably understood that this wasn't incomprehensible gibberish. I remain convinced they knew I was speaking Māori.

Yet another entry read: 'Patient was seen in room of X performing a satanic ritual.' My recollection of this incident is that there was a person who was staying in the unit who committed suicide in his room. I asked the staff if they could get one of the kaumātua (elders) into the room to do a blessing. They refused and in fact one of them said, 'That's okay. He's Catholic anyway; he's going to hell.' I realised I needed to take care of this myself. I took some water down there and I did my own karakia in that room. I thought, if these guys aren't going to do it, then I will attempt to bless this room to make it safe for the next person. I was punished for that.

Electroconvulsive Therapy

My experience was that the medications weren't working. In fact, they removed my ability to distance myself from all my tormenting voices and visions. My day consisted of sitting there, literally screaming and begging for death in my head.

Eventually the doctors started having discussions about this. I imagine they were saying, 'Well, we can't keep throwing medications at this guy. We've tried everything; it's not working.' They thought, 'Perhaps if we can in some way alter his brain patterns that might be helpful.' So they tried electroconvulsive therapy (ECT).

I received 27 doses of ECT. That's 27 times I was strapped to a table and had the national grid go through my skull. I believe the logic of this was they were trying to jump-start my brain activity. One thing I also picked up when I was going through my patient files was that when I was having ECT, it would be noted in my file which medications had been used. In most, it was noted that I had been given sedatives, which I assume were given so that I wouldn't have a full convulsion on the table. But there were a couple of instances of ECT when no sedatives were listed. Therefore, I believe I was actually given ECT without an anaesthetic. And that is certainly my memory of it. I distinctly remember being strapped down and having one of the orderlies lean over me and abuse me and tell me that unless I play the game, they were going to keep doing this. That wasn't treatment for me: that was pretty much torture. As far as I recall, the ECT had no beneficial effect for me on all the voices and visions and other experiences I was having. On the contrary, I felt much more negative and angry after that.

Following this there was another big meeting. My parents believed it was a discharge meeting, but they were wrong. At that time there was a particular part of our Mental Health Act where you could basically place someone as a ward of the state. The psychiatrist had this conversation with my parents. They weren't trying to be cruel: they were trying to be humane. They didn't want my parents to have to constantly come and visit and see me becoming more and more unwell.

I remember the doctor saying, 'Your son, Egan, your youngest boy – he's not coming home. Egan has potentially one of the worst cases of paranoid schizophrenia we've ever encountered. There is absolutely no form of treatment that can bring him back. We are going to ask you guys to please allow us to take him into our care. If, however, you choose not to allow that, we will commence legal proceedings to ensure that occurs.' I remember so clearly the look in my parents' eyes: the look of hope dying. If anything, it is probably that look that has kept me working in mental health for 20-odd years. It is the look that I don't want anyone else to have. To be told that there is no hope; there is no healing for this person.

Thankfully, my parents were not in agreement with what had been said. They battled it, and eventually I was released. One of the parting gifts I was given was my diagnosis of paranoid schizophrenia. That's always a fantastic conversation starter and conversation killer. I do find, however, it's intensely helpful when you are at a party and the last really yummy canapé is sitting there on the table and I can mention, 'Hi, my name is Egan and I'm the one with schizophrenia,' and that person is going to walk away and leave you with the canapé. So it has its advantages.

Understanding My Experiences

I was unwell on and off over a five-year period. My initial admission was for six months but adding all the other times I've been in a psychiatric ward, I have spent over two years locked up in acute psychiatric facilities. I have pretty much maintained stability from the age of 23. Although I have had plenty of difficult times, I have been back to university and completed a Bachelor of Arts in philosophy, film and television, and Māori language, and later a postgraduate qualification in management. I like to think that I have been a present husband and father to my whānau. For the last six years I have been a team coach in our region for the Pathways Trust, a national non-governmental mental health provider.

My understanding of what happened to me during those periods of unwellness is that I was experiencing both psychosis and intense spiritual experiences that overwhelmed me. It is clear to me that utilising and abusing cannabis really blew me into that place of psychosis. I have known many people who have experienced psychotic episodes and have supported friends through their own illnesses and know how scary those experiences can be for others and their whānau, as well as myself.

I consider that our mind and spirit are linked. Mental illness and spiritual distress can happen at the same time. In my case, initially there were wairua experiences which I could identify because I was aware of my Nanny and my sister with me and other perceptions I had experienced prior to smoking marijuana. I know I also had psychosis going on because I had delusional thoughts. For example, I remember 100 percent believing I could break out of the psychiatric hospital by getting a remote-controlled car and somehow putting my wairua into this car and driving it out of the ward. I was having those kinds of experiences alongside my wairua experiences.

Healing

My healing journey started after my first discharge from hospital. I returned to Tūrangi with my parents. They arranged for me to see a tohunga (Māori healer) I already knew, who was a tohunga rongoā (herbal medicine expert). He prescribed natural medicines to clean out my system. His partner was a tohunga wairua; someone who moved in the spiritual realms. She taught me the best way to use karakia to calm myself and settle what was going on for me.

Other healing elements came from my whānau, such as my experience of feeling understood by my mother. When I returned home, I had frequent conversations with her about the many things I was seeing and hearing. She always gave me the time I needed. She could explain many of my experiences, and her explanations made sense. This made me feel I wasn't alone.

I also had a feeling of forgiveness from both my parents. Immediately after my first discharge from hospital, I was acutely aware of bringing shame upon my family. Tūrangi was a very small town, and I knew word would spread in our local community that I was mentally unwell and had been locked up in a psychiatric institution. Not only this, but I felt I had gotten myself into trouble with using marijuana. I knew my parents were staunchly anti-marijuana and anti-drugs. As a nurse, my mother was very familiar with mental health problems exacerbated by marijuana. My Dad worked in local prisons and had also seen people with negative consequences from their drug use.

I used marijuana a few times after I was finally discharged from Tokanui. Each time I would become unwell, though not grossly psychotic. This was enough for me to realise that I can't touch marijuana without risking a psychotic break.

My parents never made me feel guilty or inferior for what happened. I recall my Dad coming into my room and telling me, 'Son, we are happy to have you home.' For me, that alleviation of shame was an important part of the aroha (love). I didn't need to feel whakamā. Whakamā is usually translated to mean shame but culturally it has a much deeper meaning. Whakamā literally means to turn white or pale. It's like your essence – your very soul – has been torn out of you. It can be such a damaging and deflating experience that it can render you more vulnerable to negative spiritual entities.

A further healing element was my whakapapa (genealogical connections). After my first admission, my parents told me much more about my tīpuna (ancestors). I was struck by the sheer number of them who had very similar matekite and matakite experiences to me. That helped me realise that these experiences were not an abomination but simply my inheritance.

For me, matekite refers to experiences that relate to spirits and things that have gone before us. For example, it can refer to the seeing of spiritual entities around people. Matakite refers to the future sense. It relates to things that are yet to come. For instance, sometimes I see something which I believe is about to happen in the future. To me that is matakite. There are some people who only sense spirits and some people who don't see spirits but may have experiences that help them know the future. Some people may have both. These are two different elements of spiritual experience.

As a result of hearing these stories, I began to realise that such experiences in my whānau were as ordinary as me inheriting my koro's (grandfather's) cheekbones. That was very healing for me because it relieved me of fearing I was a freak. In this context it was expected that I would have such experiences. Once it was identified when I was very young, this awareness was nurtured in me. In my teenage years, I now know how carefully my mother guided me away from illicit substances. She didn't explain her reasons at the time. However, she would have known that if I started using drugs it could overwhelm me. I was used to being immersed in a river of wairua, but as soon as I started smoking pot, it turned into an ocean. Finally, it became a tidal wave that I couldn't contain.

Distinguishing Wairua from Psychosis

I think it's important to consider which of my experiences were wairua and which were psychosis. I know that I have experienced times of both being blended. When I was recovering in Tūrangi with my folks, my mother was a huge help in ascertaining which end of that wairua-psychosis spectrum my experiences were sitting at. She was highly attuned to sensing and 'knowing' wairua. I'd let her know what I was experiencing, and she would respond with 'Oh, that's wairua, you're okay; return to what you know. Do your karakia, wear your taonga (precious pendant), go for a walk and cleanse yourself in the awa.' Sometimes she would respond with 'Yeah, that's not wairua. Focus your mind. Meditate. Let that just pass on. Kia tau, kia tau – let it settle, let it settle.'

Occasionally she might respond with, 'So these bits are wairua, they're tika (correct). Those other bits, they're teka (rubbish/psychosis).' Mum – along with the tohunga who were supporting me, particularly the female tohunga who held deep knowledge within te ao wairua (the spiritual realm) – taught me to recognise and discern the difference within my experiences. That discernment and familiarity has afforded me the ability to maintain clarity within those experiences.

Often I focus on the nuances of the combination of sensory input I am receiving to help me discern whether what I am experiencing may be wairua or hallucinations. I tend to experience wairua via three or even four of my senses, such as sight together with smell, feeling and an innate knowing. On other occasions it may be sight with hearing, taste and feeling. Depending on how immediate the experience is, I may receive input via all senses. In contrast, I tend to experience psychosis via a maximum of two senses.

My process for discerning psychosis from wairua is what I call my 'filter'. It starts with a 'ping' on one of my senses. I might initially just have a feeling, or a visual impression, a sound, a smell or a taste. However, if I focus on it, and allow that experience to wash over me, it may trigger other senses. So let's say the first perception is a voice. I would focus and wait to see what else may make itself known to me. Let's imagine the next sensory impression is a smell. Now I have two senses triggering. It may just stop there. Or else it may continue with other senses like feeling or taste or just an inexplicable knowing.

Generally, these perceptions don't all come at once but in waves that follow the initial sense that was triggered. This allows me time and space to discern its origin; to decide within myself if this is a psychotic experience or a wairua one. The 'sequential triggering' allows me to remain distanced enough to discern and thus assist in maintaining my safety within those experiences.

Even when I sense a presence there in space next to me, or nearby, I still have to use this filtering system. Often sensing a presence is a wairua experience for me. However, occasionally when I have felt such a presence, it turned out to be – from my own surmising and filtering based on additional triggering of sensory input – just paranoia; therefore, a psychotic experience.

To illustrate this process, I recall one time – and I apologise for the gross nature of this example – of going to the toilet at home in Tūrangi. To add further context, I'd been the only one home that day and hadn't been to the toilet yet. I walked into the toilet, and I saw an overflowing toilet bowl of excrement and toilet paper (visual) just bubbling out onto the toilet floor. I was also struck by the most pungent smell that made me gag (olfactory). After the initial shock of seeing and smelling this, I thought through what I was experiencing. Some aspects of it made me think it might not be real. I reasoned that unless there was some form of overflow issue in the plumbing, which had never occurred before, what I was seeing and smelling were likely to be hallucinations. I closed the toilet door, went outside, took my shoes and socks off, and stood upon the lawn to literally ground myself. I meditated and settled and silenced my mind until I felt even again. Then I went inside and opened the toilet door, and it was clean again. All I had seen and smelt prior was gone; it was never there in the first place.

Sometimes my hallucinations are indications of significant unresolved wairua matters that need to be settled and sorted out. That experience of the overflowing toilet was a catalyst that led me to consider what was going on for me on a wairua level. It prompted me to ponder about what 'shit' I had been hanging on to that might be ready to spill over. After much karakia and reflection, the answer came to me. I needed to let go of past pains: childhood abuse that would never be addressed in person because the perpetrator had passed away. The toilet experience spurred me on to release the shackles of that trauma. I had continued to carry that person's 'shit' within me. It needed to be flushed away lest it bubble up and literally stink up my life. It was theirs, not mine. That 'psychotic experience', once I could make sense of it, contributed to the start of me releasing what I had carried for decades. Later that day it occurred to me that over the morning, prior to my hallucinations, I had been ruminating on those traumatic events. I believe that 'psychotic experience' was wairua giving me a message: 'Hey you! Wake up! This is not yours. Release it. Flush it down!'

Distinguishing Post-traumatic Voices and Visions from Psychosis and Wairua

Probably the most disturbing example for me of a traumatic memory appearing as a combination of hallucinations occurred when my son was very little. I was changing his nappy and cleaning him up after many nights of broken sleep. I now realise that as a result of my lack of sleep, I was teetering on the edge. While I was changing him, I had a flashback and suddenly could see my own abuser abusing my son. I completely lost it.

I started swinging my fists at nothing but an overlaid image in my head. I was swearing like a sailor, 'Get away from my son! You …' Thankfully none of that overlay was in the vicinity of my son. However, this was one hell of a wake-up call for me. It spurred me on to sort out my trauma before it endangered my loved ones. I feel nauseous just thinking about how horrible it would have been if that 'overlay' had been over my darling son. I am so very grateful the outcome was just hitting air.

I was hearing so many voices in Tokanui I could not identify the majority of them. However, I frequently heard my abuser's voice. This voice was saying exactly what they had said when I was being abused, but also attempting to converse with and taunt me. At that point the perpetrator of my abuse was still alive and so these experiences were auditory hallucinations. This person, who was not closely connected to our family, passed away some years later, when I had returned to Tūrangi and started my healing journey. Perhaps one month after they died, that voice came back, albeit briefly. I believe it was very transient because I knew they were dead, and I was actually thankful they had died. I was thankful because now they were either a hallucination or wairua. To be honest, I wasn't sure which it was. My spiritual well-being was still relatively fresh at that time, so my ability to discern was not 100 percent. Either way I just uttered the karakia and it stopped. That voice has never returned since.

Relationship with Te Atua

My relationship with Te Atua or God is relevant here. I am comfortable with whatever names others might have for that Source. I was raised as a Roman Catholic and most of my whānau are Catholic. My Dad and later my Mum were Eucharistic ministers in our church. My mother taught me that it was important to always have that connection to divinity. She maintained that was your safety. She would say that with wairua experiences, your divine Source is your armour, and your sword if needs be as well. The most critical thing is looking after that connection. However, when I became unwell, I really felt disconnected from God. At times I believed that I was the Source, that I had all this power, that this was me. However, that was a sure sign that the opposite was the case: that I was less connected, confused and no longer protected or safe. At the same time, the high doses of antipsychotic medication I was on also made me feel distant from that connection. After leaving hospital, as my medication was reduced, even though I was still having many positive and negative voices and visions, after some time my spiritual mind became clearer. I could realise that the Source is not me; the Source is God, and I needed to reconnect with that. This was important in my recovery.

Continuing My Recovery

I'm now 50 years old. I've spent more than half my life in a process of recovery: of living towards maintaining balance with these experiences. I've not always been successful. Since the age of 23, I have had three real big relapses where I have lost touch with reality. Those were usually driven by stress. I have a terrible habit of saying yes to things I should have said no to and putting unnecessary pressure on myself. However, I haven't been institutionalised during any of these episodes. I have just managed them with the support of my family.

Wiremu

I acknowledge Egan for having the courage to share his story so that we can all learn from him. Each person's lived experience is unique to that person. What I notice about Egan's situation is that he was able to deal with very negative life experiences during his periods of unwellness and somehow transform them into something positive. I am reminded of part of a karakia, 'Tēnei te pō, nau mai te ao' (At our darkest moments, we may find the light we need) which I referred to in Chapter 2. Egan experienced some extremely dark times in his childhood and then early adult life, and somehow emerged from that. With the light that followed, he has been able to illuminate things for others.

Spiritual Doorways

Egan had a lot of matekite experiences as a tamaiti (child). Like many others, when he left home and went to university, he was affected by peer pressure and ended up smoking weed. However, due to his matekitetanga, which is everything pertaining to his gift, Egan was much more vulnerable to the effects of this substance on his spiritual attunement than other young people who are not matekite.

Marijuana heightened his perceptual awareness markedly. If we talk about ngā kūaha or doorways of understanding, I believe that marijuana opened up his spiritual doorways. As he smoked more and more, it's as if these doorways to his senses became wedged wide open. At that time, he had no ability to close them. However, for Egan, he had a number of doorways open already – like several doorways coming off the same corridor. He could see spiritual entities; he could hear things in the realm of wairua; he could pick up energy fields related to others and even discern future or past events of people he was meeting for the first time. If all these doorways became wedged open at the same time, no wonder he felt overwhelmed by all the spiritual sensory experiences he was being bombarded with. Some people may be open to just one modality, and even that could be distressing if that one doorway is opened up further. Others may have the ability to be selective about what they see or hear or allow into their space. But often young people who have skills for coping with their matekite experiences have been guided by elders and other family members.

I think it is significant that Egan became unwell at a time when he had moved away from his whānau. Prior to that, his mother was there to guide him in the realm of wairua. She would have been steering him away from hazards like marijuana. If he had any doubts about what he was experiencing, he could kōrero (speak) to her. He also had the spiritual protection from the mana of his immediate and wider whānau. When he moved away, he was less protected.

Just as using marijuana can alter the mind and open up a doorway, other conditions such as leaving home for a big city can have a similar effect. At the same time, traumatic experiences, like sexual, physical and emotional abuse, can open up spiritual doorways to negative entities and result in distressing voices and visions. A traumatic brain injury could do the same. I explain this further in Chapter 9.

Trampling on Mana

For Egan, many aspects of his psychiatric treatment were unhelpful and traumatic. It seems there was very little chance for his voice or any voice from his whānau to be heard in decision-making about his treatment. As I said in Chapter 2, when you take someone's rākau (ceremonial staff) away from them, then you remove their authority, and you risk trampling on their mana. Apart from other ill-effects, this can make someone more vulnerable to negative entities in the spiritual realm.

However, some incidents that Egan described go further than this. They demonstrate blatant disregard of his human rights. When he was doing karakia and was told to shut up, that was a violation of tapu (something sacred or forbidden). The cushion incident is another example. Being so heavily sedated had a very negative impact on his sense of self-efficacy. His experience of ECT was that it was used in an abusive fashion; he certainly wasn't consenting to it. I would consider that to be a further violation of tapu. I'm not criticising any individual psychiatrists or other clinicians for what happened to Egan, but systems that trample heavily on the mana of people do a lot of damage.

Aroha

A turning point for me in Egan's story was the moment when his whānau fought for him to come home. My hunch is that the aroha of his parents and other whānau members was a critical part of Egan's healing journey.

Aroha is often translated as love, affection or compassion. For me it goes deeper than that. 'Aro' means to give attention to something. 'Hā' refers to the breath. However, more than that, 'te hā' is the breath of life. I would say that 'te hā' is the evidence that Io (Supreme Being) is within us. When we feel aroha flowing, we have a direct connection to Te Kaihanga (The Creator). As a result, aroha is an important ingredient in healing. It is a catalyst for the restoration of tapu. Love overcomes many things.

For Egan, the love of his whānau surrounding him began to build up his resilience. It gradually re-energised him, recharging his batteries. This healing time with his whānau allowed for the restoration of tapu that had been violated at the time of his psychiatric admission, as well as earlier in his life. The restoration of tapu brings about the restoration of mana. While the restoration of his mana would have taken a long time, gradually it became more possible for Egan to take back his rākau, his spiritual authority. We are divinely connected to a source that affirms we are sacred beings. As a result, we have been given authority to be able to take charge of negative things that are impinging on our space spiritually.

Allister

Psychiatric Abuse and Institutional Racism

Even though I have read Egan's account a number of times, I still feel a mixture of emotions when I think about his narrative, especially his description of the treatment he experienced during his first prolonged psychiatric admission. I am struck by his graphic description of clinician responses which dismissed and attempted to abolish his efforts to cope with such distressing experiences using Māori practices that had sustained him in his early years. His account is a vivid illustration of the destructive colonising effect of such interactions. I feel ashamed that such abuses have been carried out in the name of psychiatry and mental health care.

Around the time that Egan had his first psychiatric admission, I qualified as a doctor and within five years had started my training in psychiatry. Egan's description of loss of mana and dignity during his treatment reminds me of a number of institutional psychiatric settings I worked in during on-call duties on evenings and weekends in the mid-1990s. While I don't recall witnessing such blatant racism and abuse as Egan experienced, I sometimes noticed coercive interactions I felt distinctly uncomfortable about, involving staff who appeared frustrated and perhaps burnt out. These situations were compounded by the whānau-unfriendly atmosphere in these institutional settings. At the same time, I also witnessed compassionate and skilled clinicians providing excellent mental health care in the same less than optimal environments.

Each of the wards I am referring to were closed over the following years during the deinstitutionalisation reforms in the mid to late 1990s. However, as Egan notes, while negative stories of people's experiences of mental health care are less common, we still have a lot more work to do to reduce coercive practices, especially in acute psychiatric hospital settings. Consumer advocate leaders such as Egan and Mary O'Hagan, a former mental health commissioner in New Zealand, have continued to highlight the need for further change, including the further development of peer-led mental health support settings (Bidois, 2017, 2019; O'Hagan, 2015).

Egan described his experiences of abuse and punishment, and the suppression of his attempts to cope with his distress by using karakia and haka and by grounding himself on the earth. His institutional care shows a clear pattern of responses that suppressed his Māori identity, language and coping style, and rendered his wairua experiences invisible.

It is often tempting to give mental health practitioners of previous eras the benefit of the doubt and assume that most had good intentions, and therefore such problematic practices were just down to a few bad apples. However, delving more carefully into the history of mental health care can be very revealing. Hilary Stace (2019), a disability researcher, has highlighted the role that eugenics theories had in the development of mental health asylums in Aotearoa, like the one Egan was admitted to. She defines eugenics as a pseudoscience based on Darwin's theory of evolution which asserted that the human race could be improved by selecting out 'undesirable' members of society, such as those with mental illness or disabilities, separating them off from their communities and attempting to prevent them from reproducing.

A group interested in these theories met and formed a Eugenics Education Society in Dunedin in 1910. This included prominent local members of the medical community such as Truby King (Stace, 2019). King is most widely known as founder of the Plunket Society in New Zealand, an organisation set up to attend to the wellbeing of mothers and babies. He was also medical superintendent of Seacliff Mental Asylum, near Dunedin in the South Island, and later head of the Department of Mental Hospitals, the central government department responsible for all the mental hospitals in New Zealand. Theodore Gray, a Scottish medical practitioner who succeeded King in this national psychiatric administration role, was another strong advocate for eugenics policies. He proposed segregated villa-style accommodation for mental hospitals on rural properties, and compulsory sterilisation for those with intellectual disabilities and mental illness (Stace, 2019).

Although such sterilisation practices were eventually rejected, in 1928 the Mental Defectives Amendment Act legalised the compulsory removal of children with disabilities from their families and their subsequent placement in institutional care. Hilary Stace (2019) has pointed out that Māori families were much more severely affected by such policies due to the added impact of racism and colonisation. This is the historical backdrop to Egan's psychiatrists suggesting to his whānau that Egan would be better off in institutional care, even when his treatment was so evidently ineffective.

For me, as a Pākehā (New Zealand European) psychiatrist, it is painful to reflect on these unjust practices in mental health settings in New Zealand. However, we need to know our history in order to see the patterns clearly and ensure that these injustices can be addressed. For example, there is clear evidence that Māori are disproportionately affected by the use of seclusion practices in mental health settings in New Zealand (McLeod et al., 2017). The history of racist responses to Māori in mental health care is an important part of understanding the context to that complex problem. Since 2012, the Ministry of Health in New Zealand has prioritised the reduction and elimination of the use of seclusion and restraint for Māori and non-Māori in mental health care settings (Ministry of Health, 2012).

It is a cruel irony that, at the exact time Egan was experiencing his first hospitalisation at Tokanui, during which his Māori values and culture were derided and suppressed, New Zealand's first bicultural mental health unit was running in the *same* institution. In that setting, Egan may have had a markedly different response from Māori staff. Mental health care in large institutions has been criticised throughout the history of such care. Erving Goffman, who studied asylum care in the 1950s in the United States, identified practices and processes that could cause people who were compelled to stay in institutions to lose hope, identity and sense of self (Chow & Priebe, 2013).

In the last 20 years, young adults presenting with distressing symptoms resembling psychosis in Aotearoa would commonly be seen in community-based Early Intervention Services (Theuma et al., 2007). These services focus on engaging with young people in the context of their families, and aim to offer multifaceted care approaches which may include: family therapy; support in returning to education or work; psychological therapies such as trauma work; support for Māori whānau from Māori cultural workers; and physical treatments such as medication. Admission to hospital is reserved for people who present with much more severe symptoms and are at clear risk to themselves or others. There is greater acknowledgement in these services that addressing the symptoms and problems people are facing is more important than focusing on which specific diagnosis may explain the person's predicament. For young people with hallucinations, other psychotic symptoms, drug use and trauma in their background, clarifying diagnoses can sometimes help but may have limited utility in guiding treatment (Maj, 2018; McGorry, 2015). Despite recent developments in trauma-informed care, we have a long way to go to provide optimal trauma-informed assessment of people with hallucinations and other psychosis-like symptoms, and to provide effective and timely trauma therapies such as Eye Movement Desensitization and Reprocessing (EMDR) and Trauma-Focused Cognitive Behaviour Therapy (TF-CBT) (van den Berg et al., 2015).

In addition to the above changes, there has been wide acknowledgement of the need for culturally appropriate approaches for Māori people in mental health care (Durie, 1998). One example is the adolescent inpatient psychiatry facility in my local area of Porirua, which was set up as a bicultural unit with kaumātua as part of the team. Practices such as use of mihimihi (greeting speeches), karakia and waiata (songs) make this a more hospitable environment for Māori young people. However, alongside these positive developments, there are very few situations in which Māori healing consultations would be offered alongside other conventional approaches in early intervention for psychosis assessment and care.

In my view, the most important development in mental health services in Aotearoa in the last 20 years has been employing people with lived experience of mental distress in mental health teams. These colleagues have gradually challenged taken-for-granted processes, practices and ways of talking about mental health and unwellness. Their presence has encouraged improvements in mental health practices and culture in those teams fortunate enough to have them (Scholz et al., 2017).

Use of Electroconvulsive Therapy

I also wish to comment on Egan's experience of electroconvulsive therapy (ECT). I was appalled to learn about Egan's experience of being given ECT without anaesthetic. I had heard reports of such abusive practices two decades earlier (Stace, 2019), but not as recently as the early 1990s. In 2001, New Zealand Prime Minister Helen Clark apologised to patients who had been subjected to the abusive use of ECT as a punishment and without anaesthetic while being treated as children at Lake Alice Hospital in the 1970s, in the Whanganui region (Stace, 2019). Egan's description of ECT being used by staff in a coercive and abusive way has also been reported by others, for example, people whose experiences were described in the Department of Internal Affairs 2007 report, *Te Āiotanga: Report of the Confidential Forum for Former In-Patients of Psychiatric Hospitals*. Clearly many people, in a wide range of psychiatric institutions over many years, were severely affected by these unacceptable and abusive practices.

Alongside these facts, as a psychiatrist I am also aware of clear evidence that ECT can be an effective and humane treatment for some people with the most severe and distressing mental illnesses (Sackeim, 2017). These can include catatonia, acute psychosis, and severe depression. In some instances, a person can be so unwell that they may not be eating or drinking. In others, medications may not have been helpful, or the side effects of medication may have been unacceptable. In addition, modern ECT methods have resulted in fewer ECT side effects (Sackeim, 2017).

ECT has not been part of my practice as a community child and adolescent psychiatrist in the last two decades. Other therapies and treatments are effective and more appropriate for young people who seek our assistance. However, early in my career, as a first-year trainee in psychiatry in Lower Hutt in 1995, my duties included participating in ECT treatment: helping prepare adult patients for this procedure; discussing the potential benefits and possible negative effects with them; seeking their consent; and participating during their treatment and recovery. My supervisor, the consultant psychiatrist on our ward, was present before, during and after the procedure. A consultant anaesthetist was present throughout the procedure to make sure that the anaesthesia was carried out to a high standard. I recall conversations between the anaesthetist and my supervisor about which anaesthetic agents caused fewer side effects and which methods of carrying out ECT treatment would minimise negative effects.

During this time, I recall meeting a 50-year-old man who was becoming severely depressed and was tormented by distressing voices. As I was arranging for him to be admitted to hospital, he told me that the only treatment that worked well for him in this situation was ECT. He relaxed considerably when he learnt that this treatment would be available to him. During ECT his condition improved rapidly, and he made a good recovery.

It is obvious that in the early 1990s there were ECT practices in other New Zealand settings that fell far below the standards that are used today. Poor standard of care is deplorable, but abusive use of procedures such as ECT is completely unacceptable. The context of care and the quality of the therapeutic relationship is critical here. Trusting relationships with clinicians, whānau involvement and shared decision-making processes, can lead to a very different outcome from Egan's experience. A surgical incision without anaesthetic and without consent would be considered a horrific assault, but can be welcome and lifesaving when given with appropriate anaesthesia and in circumstances in which you understand the purpose and procedure, have given your consent and trust your surgical team. I consider ECT in a similar light. It is understandable that negative perceptions of ECT persist after historical abuse in institutional care and negative depictions in mainstream media. And for Egan it was clearly traumatic and ineffective.

Lived Experience

The views of people with lived experience of mental distress on the meaning of voices and visions have been ignored throughout most of the history of psychiatry and psychology. In recent years this state of affairs has begun to change. Increasing numbers of authors with lived experience have critiqued and questioned psychiatric theories on voices and visions (Bidois, 2017; Coleman, 1999; Gutkovich, 2020; Longden, 2010; O'Hagan, 2015). Dillon and May (2002) have argued that clinical interactions frequently devalue people's own views about their voices and visions and degrade the meanings they put on them. They maintain that people can recover when they have an opportunity to reclaim their experiences from the narrow confines of psychiatric interpretations and choose narratives that make most sense to them. They contend that a sense of personal agency combined with a narrative that feels coherent is much more enabling than being the passive recipient of a 'brain fault' hypothesis from your psychiatrist.

Dillon and May advocate for hearing voices groups in which people can connect with others with similar experiences. By sharing stories of struggle and hope, people can free themselves from isolation, self-criticism and shame, and rediscover their own sense of expertise in their lives (Dillon & May, 2002). In such groups, people can hear about a much wider range of meaning frameworks. Many attest to the significance of adversity early in their lives and how understanding that can help in making sense of voices and visions (Longden, 2010; Coleman, 1999). Other frameworks include socio-political and spiritual meaning systems (Dillon & May, 2002). Longden et al. (2018) carried out a systematic study of the impact of Hearing Voices Network self-help groups and highlighted the benefits of these groups in reducing isolation, enhancing feelings of safety and recovery, and facilitating coping with voices.

Challenges and Questions for Mental Health Care

The consumer movement has played a very important role in scrutinising psychiatric practice and calling for change. At the same time, over several decades Māori leaders have highlighted the importance of Māori identity for the wellbeing of individuals and whānau, and the need for this to be addressed in mental health care (Durie, 1998; Kingi et al., 2017; NiaNia et al., 2017; Rangihuna et al., 2018). Despite this, the matters that Egan raises about recognition of matekite experiences and their complex interrelationship with psychotic illness remain frequently overlooked in psychiatry in Aotearoa. Given the silencing and ignoring of Māori and other Indigenous perspectives on the meanings of voices and visions, and the colonising effects of care in mental health facilities over generations, how can those of us in the mental health field respond? If we assume that Egan's experience is not unique, are there any steps we can take to address these injustices?

One possible pathway forward could involve allocating research resources to careful study of some of the questions raised by Egan's experiences and the interpretations he and Wiremu put on them. In the past, researching wairua may have been dismissed by mental health researchers as unscientific. In addition, Māori communities and their elders may well have been reluctant to participate, given the possibility that sacred matters could be disrespected, desecrated or misappropriated, and subjected to the harsh and colonising gaze of Pākehā academic scrutiny.

Given Egan's narrative and Wiremu's korero in previous chapters, it appears obvious that Māori have suffered in mainstream mental health services as a result of Māori understandings being overlooked and sidelined in psychiatry. Linda Tuhiwai Smith has pointed out that a decolonising approach to mental health research would prioritise Māori paradigms and concerns (Smith, 2012). A kaupapa Māori (Māori-centred) research method would have Māori leadership and authority to determine Māori priorities and purposes.

I'm not sure what research questions might be a focus for Māori researchers. However, here are some of my own questions as a result of reading Egan's story.

Could people who have matekite experiences and later go on to develop distressing voices and visions be suffering from spiritual distress rather than a psychiatric problem? What about those, such as Egan, who are matekite and then later develop severe and distressing voices and visions, but in addition have other signs of psychosis such as delusions or disorganised thinking? If they appear to meet criteria for a psychotic illness like schizophrenia but then don't respond to psychiatric treatment, what are we missing here? Is it possible that they may have different healing and treatment needs due to their spiritual awareness? Are people who have matekite experiences more prone to distressing perceptual experiences if they use cannabis heavily? Is it possible to reliably identify people who have enhanced spiritual awareness and who are also experiencing symptoms that suggest they have a psychotic illness, to examine whether they respond differently to various treatments, including antipsychotic medication, compared to other people with psychotic disturbances who are not spiritually aware? What were the therapeutic approaches used by Egan's whānau and tohunga that helped him on his path to recovery, and could these approaches help other young Māori with matekite and psychotic symptoms after using cannabis? Egan states that his whānau have successfully helped him through at least three major relapses without requiring hospitalisation: how did they do that? What resources would a whānau require to similarly support their family member through such a profoundly distressing episode? I am interested to know what Egan would suggest for how such research endeavours might proceed.

Finally, in reflecting on the significance of Egan's story, I wonder if the most important contribution may not be the challenges and questions he raises for psychiatry and mental health care, but the hope his story may offer others who find themselves facing such dark times in their lives. New Zealand writer, poet and researcher Karlo Mila has expressed this much better than I could:

> If you do find yourself in that frightening terrain … the last thing you feel is that someone else, someone wise, someone wonderful, someone brave, someone beautiful, has been here before me. There are so few signposts, clues, crumbs, that show that – not only has someone smart been here before you – but that survivor, that person has left a crumb trail behind, to lead you, to reassure you, to remind you, that there is a way out.
>
> (Mila-Schaaf, 2010)

Egan

It is interesting for me to read Wiremu and Allister's responses to my recollections and to reflect on their different perspectives. Similar to Wiremu, I view wairuatanga (the spiritual dimension) as a foundation of strength for us as Māori. To separate ourselves from our wairua is to separate ourselves from our sense of power. Wairua goes beyond the physical and will still exist when the physical body starts giving up. However, it's still important to take care of our physical well-being. Mental health clinicians and wairua practitioners have a lot to offer each other. These kinds of partnerships can help create more appropriate services.

Partnerships

So how can clinicians and others best help people like me who may be suffering from psychotic illness and spiritual distress at the same time? How can we tell the difference between someone who is suffering from spiritual distress that looks like psychosis and psychosis that looks like spiritual distress? I believe this is why we need psychiatrists and other clinicians, like Allister, and tohunga, like Papa Wiremu, working together within mental health services. When someone is in distress, it can be very helpful to have both sets of eyes on their situation. I don't believe in polarised positions. I know some people might say, 'It's all psychiatry' and others say, 'It's all wairua'. None of that is helpful. People don't exist on the edges; they exist somewhere floating in the middle. Working together will be beneficial, not only for the people they see and their families but also for the wairua practitioners and clinicians themselves. It will offer an opportunity to understand each other better and gain a deeper respect for each other. For some time, it has been an us versus them situation. If we want people to heal, we have to work as a 'we'.

My mother's view was that it was possible to work with all these different perspectives. When I asked her how she balanced her spiritual experiences with her roles as psychiatric nurse and Eucharistic minister, her response was that she saw no disconnect between each of these viewpoints. She was convinced that her wairua experiences came from God. She also believed that her training in psychiatric nursing was gifted from God so that she could help people who were lost in those places. Not only that but she viewed her role as a Catholic Eucharistic minister as an opportunity to serve God. She maintained that if she had been Muslim or any other religion, it would have been just the same.

For clinicians, to distinguish psychosis from matekite experiences I would recommend having someone like Papa Wiremu alongside you. I am totally in support of the idea that tohunga should be employed in mental health services alongside other clinicians. At the same time, I would advise caution. There needs to be rigour behind it. Just as with medicine, having appropriate registering bodies for tohunga will be important. There are some people who would purport to be skilled wairua practitioners when they are not. When someone is claiming to be matekite, I would be asking: Where is the whakapapa of this in their whānau? These abilities don't magically appear out of nowhere. They are generally inherited and there will be people in their whānau that came before with similar wairua gifts. What defines a tohunga is whether your people put you as such. It's like anything within Māori culture; it's the people that place you in those roles. They are the ones that give you those roles, and they are the ones who will take you out of those roles if you in any way use them wrongly. If you don't consult tohunga with appropriate expertise, then you can have a situation such as that which happened in Wainuiomata in 2007, where a simple blessing turned into a young woman being drowned (Otago Daily Times, 2010). A little knowledge can be dangerous.

Research

Allister raised some suggestions about research. There is a definite need for more Māori research in this area. I believe Māori researchers are more likely to understand such experiences, but collaboration with non-Māori can be helpful in bringing the findings to a wider audience and may help influence others such as Pākehā clinicians. In clinical work as well as research, partnerships between Māori healing and psychiatry can contribute to a balanced approach.

Marijuana

A further matter that both Allister and Wiremu referred to was the role of marijuana in my initial illness. In the early stages, the effect of the marijuana was deceptive when it appeared to be helping me. In looking back, my interpretation of this relates to my belief in good and evil. I believe that evil can be a trickster. It is capable of making you feel better in order to gain more influence over you. My mother also believed I was being tricked through my marijuana usage when I started to believe I needed to use more. By the time I realised my mistake, it was too late as I had walked into something that I wasn't ready for. In this light, Wiremu's comment about wedging the doors open through the use of marijuana made a lot of sense to me. Various elements of what I was experiencing meant I couldn't close the door on it anymore.

When I asked my mother how she made sense of me ignoring her advice about marijuana, her response was, 'That was your path.' She maintained my destiny was set before I was born. It was necessary for me to reach those dark spaces so I could recognise darkness. Emerging from that darkness had to happen in order that I might know how to bring others out. That path would give me the passion that I needed, that constant commitment to never ever give up; to advocate and fight for change so others could be spared mental health treatment experiences like that. She told me she had faith I would get through safely, and whenever her faith wavered, she would turn to karakia. During those moments she was reassured by her tīpuna that this was my journey, and I would get through it.

Connections

I view my wellbeing as being like a spider in a spider web. My wairua, my spiritual being, is like the spider, and my mauri or life force is the web. Connections extending out attach to solid elements in my life such as my whānau, whenua (land) and Source. For me to stay well, my mauri has to be strong. These connections must be healthy. When I start to experience psychosis, I become disconnected. As each string of my mauri, my web, gets cut, that web gets a little weaker. As more strands snap and others pop off, before long, just like the spider, I find myself dangling precariously by only a few threads. If any wind comes up, I can get pinged around all over the place. Over the years when my life was out of balance, I now realise I had disconnected myself from friends and whānau and from my connection to whenua. I had lost touch with the various ways I sustain my wellbeing. I believe I disconnected myself from God and stopped doing my karakia. All those bits and pieces of disconnection gradually started wearing me down, and I became fragile. Then, if a sharp gust of wind buffeted me, my experiences could start to become more disturbing. It was harder for me to stand up to them and maintain my equanimity.

What helps me regain and maintain my wellbeing is a fundamental understanding that my connections with people, places and Te Atua help my spiritual self to stay strong through everything that is coming my way.

For me, one of the defining points about whether it's psychosis or wairua is to understand: how is that person living? Is that person able to maintain a good life? Are they able to do things relatively normally but within these experiences, so that they are not so much a prisoner of them? I think that when you are matekite and you are aware of it and you have learned how to manage it and how to maintain balance, it is possible to experience a whole lot more of it and still keep your equilibrium.

People have asked me: if there was a medication that you could take that would make all your experiences stop, would you take it? My answer is no. I would not take it. These experiences are who I am. Even though these experiences are sometimes not pretty. Sometimes, as I walk through town, I can sense painful things in the lives of people I don't know as I walk past. I can feel physical pain on them from illnesses that are ailing them. I tend to see demonic entities as well, and little creatures in the wairua that crawl and scuttle. Despite the unsettling nature or even the horror of some experiences, I wouldn't shut them out. I consider that the dark side of the moon. I don't just see and hear bad stuff; I see and hear really, really good stuff as well. I want to keep the good stuff, so I won't take that pill. I won't push that magic button that is going to shut it all off. Because I don't just see demons; I see angels as well.

Kaitiaki

Our boy wasn't sleeping. He was young and we were first-time parents. We would hear this horrific terrified scream and we would run into his room to check on him. He would appear petrified and shaking. I would have this sense that something had been in his room. I ended up blessing his room a number of times. However, at that time I was so angry that some spirit had been messing with our boy that I doubt I was in the right space of mind to do a blessing. I spoke to Papa Wiremu. He suggested I hand it over to the angels to deal with. He said to do my karakia and hand it over. So, I did that. The following night my wife and I were fast asleep. In the early hours of the morning, I woke up. As I roused myself and sat up in bed, I became aware of light glowing in our corridor. My wife woke up shortly after, just in time to witness this great big golden pillar of light drifting past our door. I reassured her, 'It's okay; it's just an angel coming in to help.' After that moment, our son slept very soundly. The sense I got was that the pillar of light was very familiar. I think it was the same male angel that came to me when I was three. I think he was sent to intervene this time as well. If you were to ask me who sent him, I wouldn't be able to answer that in any definite way. However, I would assume this apa or angel is connected to our whakapapa; a kaitiaki for our whānau.

This experience reminds me of the following whakatauākī (proverb): Pae mua, pae tata, pae tawhiti. Pae mua speaks to me of taonga: abilities in wairua or gifts such as te reo (Māori language) and tikanga (customs) that have been passed down to us by those who came before. Pae tata refers to using, treasuring and safeguarding such gifts for those we have close to us now. Pae tawhiti tells us that these taonga are ultimately for the betterment of those who are yet to come. This whakatauākī is about whakapapa and continuity. It links me to this knowledge of karakia, of wairua relationships and of interventions passed down to keep us and those around us safe.

I believe in every generation there is someone like me. Once I have passed on, there will be someone in our children's generation with that spiritual awareness, and someone in their children's generation, and so on. In this story, I believe the same kaitiaki offered this gift of protection to me as a three-year-old, and then to my son and our whānau 30 years later. Our kaitiaki have this surprising ability to transcend time and space, linking us person to person with our forebears and those who are yet to come.

Notes

1 Much of Egan Bidois' story in this chapter has been taken from a transcript of the Angels and Demons episode of the 'Stuff' podcast series 'Out of My Mind: True stories about mental health, told by people who've been there', produced by Adam Dudding and first broadcast in August 2019 (Bidois, 2019).
2 Comedy duo from North America known for their appreciation of marijuana.
3 Māori cultural ritual with energetic rhythmical actions and words embodying a mana enhancing expression of identity and unity.

6 Tohu

Wiremu NiaNia, Tohu, Tai Elkington, Peter Cowley, Allister Bush, and David Epston

E kore e mōnehunehu te pūmahara	Let us not forget
Mō ngā momo rangatira o neherā	Those who came before us
Nā rātou i toro te nukuroa	They reach out to us across the vastness
O te Moana-nui-a-Kiwa me Papatūānuku	of the oceans and the earth
Ko ngā tohu o ō rātou tapuwai e	Their footsteps are etched forever
i kākahutia i runga i te mata o te whenua	across the face of the earth
He taonga, he tapu	Symbols of sacredness
He taonga, he tapu...i	

Wiremu explains the above chant as honouring those who have gone before us and paved the way.

> It is about our Māori ancestors, but in a broader sense we can take it as an acknowledgement of other Indigenous traditions from across Te Moana-nui-a-Kiwa (the Pacific Ocean) that resonate with our own ways.
>
> When we as Māori introduce ourselves, we talk about our places of belonging. We specify where our mountain is, where our rivers are, our homes, and where our people come from. We then refer to our living relationships with our ancestors. These connections are for me the essence of my identity and my wairua (spiritual wellbeing).

The importance of ancestral connection is illustrated by Tohu's story.

At 36, Tohu began experiencing severe depression and anxiety. He struggled to sleep, distanced himself from his family and felt suicidal. Tohu was referred to Te Whare Mārie, where he and support worker Tai Elkington had a session with Wiremu and community psychiatrist Dr Peter Cowley. During this session, Wiremu became aware of a Māori rangatira (leader) standing behind Tohu.

DOI: 10.4324/9781003187042-6

Sometimes seeing or hearing an ancestor can be such a vivid experience that people wonder if they might be hallucinating. This is especially likely for those who are unfamiliar with te ao wairua (the spiritual realm). Nonetheless, visitations from tīpuna (ancestors) are accepted wairua experiences in te ao Māori (the Māori world).

Tohu's story illustrates a wairua experience with a healing purpose. The narrative is told from the perspectives of Tohu, Tai, Peter, Wiremu and Allister. Tohu explains the impact this encounter had on the direction his life was taking at that time, and gives an update nine years later. The chapter begins with Tohu's account of the experiences that led up to his first session at Te Whare Mārie.

Tohu

I'm 45 now, and I must have been about 36 when my life fell apart. At the time I figured it was because of my relationship breaking up. I was taking a lot of drugs and partying with the boys all the time. Around Christmas that year I began to have difficulties sleeping. I've always been a bit of an insomniac, but then it got much worse. That was the start of everything.

I became really depressed. Over four or five weeks, the more I went down, the steeper the slope got. Before long I was suicidal. I was out of work and distanced myself from my family. I was making a dishonest living to survive. I was staying in bed for long periods and not taking care of myself. I couldn't be bothered facing the world. I would knock myself out with booze and drugs when I couldn't bear it anymore. I felt utterly hopeless.

I felt like I was circling around a black hole, just ready to fall into it. One day I was at home, deep in this hole, no longer speaking to anyone. My brother became very alarmed and rang the police. Six cops bundled me into their car and took me down to the police station.

Before long I was referred to a doctor at Te Whare Mārie. I wouldn't say I was happy to see a doctor, but I was interested in discreetly seeking help. I knew I needed something, but I wasn't sure what it was. At the time I had mean anxiety. There were moments when I would be in the supermarket and man, I just had to get out of there. This was a new experience for me. Normally I wouldn't give a hoot what anyone thought of me. So in this first meeting I was listening as the psychiatrist began asking me some questions and Tai, a support worker, was there. My anxiety was also there. I was wary. I was wondering, 'Oh yeah, what's going on here? What are these guys up to?' But at the same time I was thinking, 'Nah, this could be all right. These people are just doing their job.'

A little while later Wiremu joined us. I had never met him before. He introduced himself briefly, but then just sat quietly while Dr Peter asked me some more questions. It was sometime later when Wiremu spoke up.

I remember him saying, 'Oh, can I just interrupt? Because, bro, I can see someone standing behind you.'

Tai

I remember the session clearly. Our social worker was supposed to attend this first assessment appointment with Tohu but was unable to make it. In her absence she asked me to provide cultural support for Tohu and requested that Wiremu, our cultural therapist, attend, but without explaining why. I had spoken to Wiremu only long enough to remind him of the time, the venue and Tohu's name.

At the outset, Peter and I agreed that I would open our hui (meeting). Accordingly, I stood to acknowledge Tohu and Peter and, with Tohu's permission, started the session with a karakia (prayer). After initiating a round of introductions, I sat back while Peter introduced himself. I had noticed Tohu's stature as we greeted each other for the first time in the waiting room. He was well over six foot and solidly built. Now I had a chance to observe his attire more closely. He was dressed in shorts and gumboots and was wearing a loose-fitting T-shirt. He looked a bit rough, as if he hadn't been paying much heed to his appearance. Even though he seemed to be reluctant to be there, I didn't feel at all threatened by his demeanour. Tohu sat there unsmiling, facing Peter and me. He seemed reserved, as if he was sizing up the situation. He gave matter-of-fact answers to Peter's questions, brief and often merely yes or no. Still, he made it clear that he was wanting answers to help him make sense of his predicament. It was a little while later that Wiremu entered the room. After excusing himself for being late, and introducing himself to Tohu, he sat back and encouraged Peter and Tohu to continue their conversation.

Peter

Even though this session took place nine years ago, it stands out very clearly in my mind. In my role as a community psychiatrist at Te Whare Mārie, I was approaching this as a general assessment of someone I hadn't met before. Tai was there to provide cultural support to Tohu, and there had been prior discussion that I wasn't party to in which Wiremu had been invited to join the session as well. I was fine about that, however, Wiremu and I had not seen patients together before, and we didn't have a chance to confer before the session commenced.

I would commonly meet people who are uncomfortable about seeing a psychiatrist, and I recall that Tohu was moderately uneasy about having such a mental health conversation. The dialogue was just between us initially and after some time I sensed that he was starting to engage a little.

Nevertheless, I was having to work hard to get even minimal responses from him. It wasn't a free-flowing conversation by any means. Meanwhile Wiremu had joined us and was sitting quietly; his eyes were just drifting around the place like he was aware of what was being said but not totally concerned about being part of it.

Suddenly, partway through the interview, Wiremu sat forward and cut straight across the conversation. In a loud, firm voice, he announced that there was a Māori warrior standing behind Tohu who was connected to his whakapapa (genealogy). His tone and body language made it clear that this was highly significant. Just as he made this forceful interjection, Wiremu's eyes were totally fixated on a point just behind Tohu, as if he was watching this character on a screen. Listening to his vivid description, I imagined he was seeing a young Māori warrior, with facial tattoos, wearing a headband, perhaps even brandishing a taiaha (long wooden Māori weapon). The manner of his description was so detailed that I was convinced that he was absolutely seeing that. At no point did I have any sense that Wiremu was doing this to impress me or to unnerve me, nor to impress Tohu. Overall, it was an emphatic statement, leaving no room for any doubt whatsoever.

Having delivered this slam dunk, Wiremu then sat back in his chair. From my memory of it, that was all that he had to say. I was quite taken aback. As I waited, hoping Wiremu would elaborate further, I was thinking 'What the heck do we do now?' Wiremu's intervention felt extremely significant. I wanted to defer to Wiremu's wisdom and experience to decide how he wanted to proceed. But it seemed as if he was finished. My impression of Tohu at that moment was that he looked somewhat unnerved, but curious rather than shocked. He was unsettled in his chair. His eyes moved from Wiremu to me, perhaps not quite sure to whom he should respond. In the silence that followed I surmised that Wiremu was waiting for us to pick up where we had left off. After that dramatic interlude, it was quite difficult to get back to the psychiatric enquiry. However, I began to ask Tohu some more questions.

Wiremu

Following my late arrival in the room, and after briefly introducing myself to Tohu, I sat back to listen as Peter continued with his questions. It was sometime later that instinctively I became aware there was someone just behind Tohu. Tohu was seated near the wall and just behind his right shoulder there was a calendar. Against the blank page of the calendar, I could very clearly see the face of a Māori man. This gentleman wasn't just a still picture; he was moving before my eyes. I could see his facial features, his hair was brownish grey, and he looked at me for a moment. He was blinking and his eyes were moving. He looked alive, but I knew that others wouldn't be able to see him. What was most striking about his appearance was his mataora or full facial Māori tattoo. I knew intuitively that this was a man of distinction. I could feel his considerable mana. He was clearly a rangatira. Only someone of significance would have a mataora like that. I assumed immediately that he was a leader; perhaps a warrior. He felt ancient, as if he was someone from te ao tawhito – times of old.

My first reaction was one of respect. I felt humbled. I sat forward in my chair. While I was surprised to see him, I was also curious. I knew such a rangatira would only appear for a purpose. Soon after, I became aware of the identity of this man before me. I declared, 'Excuse me for interrupting, but there is a gentleman standing behind you, Tohu. Are you related to … ?' and I provided the name of this ancient rangatira.

Tohu sat back in his chair in surprise, staring at me. He had no immediate response to my question. His gaze moved away and after some moments of silence, he confirmed that he had a direct ancestral connection to the rangatira I had enquired about. Satisfied with that piece of information, I sat back in my chair. I wanted Peter to have the opportunity to complete his assessment process, and I knew that Tai and I would need to arrange a further time to meet with Tohu to help him make more sense of what had transpired. I knew that this tipuna (ancestor) had appeared behind Tohu in order to support him, reaffirm his connection with his whakapapa and assist him with his quandary about his identity and the predicament he was facing.

I am often surprised when wairua makes its presence felt suddenly. Even though I expect the unexpected, and I am open to anything that may eventuate, on the day of Peter's interview with Tohu I had no warning prior to the appearance of Tohu's tipuna in front of me. I had never met Tohu before that day, and I had no knowledge of his iwi (tribe) or whakapapa before entering the room. In addition, there was no kōrero (discussion) about Tohu's ancestry in my hearing in the first part of Peter's interview.

At the moment I saw this figure behind Tohu, I knew I needed to comment on the presence of this remarkable rangatira. After asking Tohu if he was related to this person, I then sat back to allow Peter to continue.

I am always careful about tikanga (protocol). In my view, Peter, as a doctor, is a rangatira with the mana (authority) that goes with that status. Tikanga demanded that I respect Peter's process related to his psychiatric interview. I didn't volunteer any information about what I had seen because I would only do that if I was invited to do so. I am always open to sharing my understanding of te ao Māori with anybody. However, having already cut across Peter's interview with my question for Tohu, I didn't want to intrude further unless Peter requested that. At the end of the interview, I knew that it would be important to meet up with Tohu soon to help him make sense of what I had seen, and I could tell that he was interested to do so. Therefore, I indicated to him that Tai and I would be in contact soon about a time to meet up.

After the Session

Even after the interview, I would have been happy to kōrero with Peter if he had approached me. However, I prefer not to impose my worldviews on other people, and so I will always wait to be invited to share my experiences and views. As it happened, I left the service nine months later. During that time, Tai and I had a number of conversations about Tohu's situation and our mahi (work) with him.

At the moment I saw Tohu's ancestor and became aware of his identity, I recognised his name but had very little knowledge of him. Over the following weeks, I did some research by consulting friends and relations who knew the history of Tohu's iwi. I learnt much more about the life story of his ancestor, who walked the earth at least 14 generations ago.

Following that initial session, Tai and I saw Tohu on several further occasions. We met with him at the beach, had kai (food) with him and gave him an opportunity to kōrero some more about what this appearance of his tipuna meant for him. He was excited about going back to learn more about his whakapapa. It was clear to me that something important changed for him during that time. After some weeks, his mood was improving and there was no more talk about suicide. He seemed to have a purpose and knew what he wanted to do next. He began to return to his whenua (land) and spent time with his whānau (family) there.

Tohu

Spiritual Protection

Wiremu said, 'There's a Māori man standing behind you, but he's not just any Māori; he's a Māori of significant standing.' Then he described him. I can't recall all the details of Wiremu's description now, but I was left with an impression of a very tall Māori character behind me, well over seven foot [2.1 metres] tall, because I'm six foot five [1.98 metres] myself. I imagined him dressed in a piupiu (flax garment), wielding a taiaha.

This news was totally unexpected. It took me some time to gather my thoughts. My biggest shock was who Wiremu saw rather than the idea that someone was there.

I distinctly remember that moment. Wiremu was dressed in a grey top. He leaned towards me as he spoke with a lot of authority about what he was seeing. Even though I'd never met Wiremu before, there was something very clear about him, as if he was there with us and nowhere else. He seemed very natural, as though he had nothing to hide. He was very open about what he was describing, suggesting to me this was an everyday thing for him. I had a strong feeling that he knew what he was talking about. Given that he made no effort to reassure me, I sensed he knew I had an inkling something was there.

After that session I had a feeling of relief. I thought back on moments in the past when I had experienced something I couldn't understand and had asked myself, 'Are you loopy?' Wiremu's observation confirmed that I wasn't loopy; I just didn't realise what was happening spiritually. Even though I still don't understand it fully, I trust it more now. As he was talking, I began to think back on puzzling moments in my life and some things started to click into place.

I often have the impression of some presence accompanying me, particularly when I am on the road, driving at night. I don't see or hear anything. I am just aware of something slightly behind me. Until that moment with Wiremu, I could never put it into words or understand it. Sometimes as I drive towards streetlights, they blow out: boom, boom, boom, one after the other. And after I drive past them, I look in the mirror and they come back on again, in the same sequence. Sometimes I've pointed it out to friends, and we've wondered about it. I've always thought it was weird but never been afraid of it. I've frequently felt I had some sort of protection. And that moment with Wiremu made me realise that it was something Māori.

An example of this protection took place one night when a friend and I were driving north to Auckland in my 4WD. At about two in the morning, we came around a corner, hit some ice and the ute started pirouetting. The instant we lost control I thought, 'Shit, we're gonna crash!' Then, to my surprise, I felt a wave of calm settle over me. It was like someone had flicked a switch. For some reason the ute didn't roll, and it just sort of straightened up, and I thought, 'What the heck happened there?'

On other occasions I have felt protected in moments of confrontation. One night in my early 30s, at a bar with friends, I was collecting some drinks and was approached by a big guy who made a menacing comment and gesture. When I responded with a light-hearted comment, he threatened me as I moved past to get back to my table. I was caught off-guard and immediately searched my mind for some connection with a previous conflict. Before I knew it there were five guys converging on me in an intimidating way and I was thinking, 'Oh shit, this isn't going to go well.' But for some unexplained reason they looked at me and hesitated and the situation just dissolved in a way that was hard to explain. This kind of thing has happened to me other times.

The earliest time I can recall a sense of being protected was when I was four years old. My Mum was working and had arranged for my younger brother and me to stay with a new babysitter. After Nan, my Dad's Mum, dropped us off, I distinctly recall realising that it didn't feel right. It didn't feel like we were in danger, but I didn't feel at all comfortable being there. I was looking out the window and thinking, 'Come on, Nan, come and get us. I wanna get out of here.' But it wasn't like normal thoughts. I was calling out to her in my mind. A little while later Nan's brown Holden pulled up. Because of my age I didn't understand exactly how it happened, but my hunch now is that something about the wairua was protective. There was something special in the connection between Nan and me, perhaps some sort of telepathic connection that explained her showing up so soon to pick us up.

When I think about it now, I realise that on my Nan's side there is an element of something spiritual running through the whole family. Even though she passed away some years ago, I still believe I have that protection from her. I have a similar feeling about my Nan on my Mum's side.

Things were not always easy in my early years. My Dad was in a gang, and he had a feisty and aggressive style. Growing up he often told me to 'toughen up'. I was expected to be staunch and masculine. There was little communication or openness between us. Anything I truly felt, I had to suppress. A number of times I saw my Mum being beaten. Dad would intimidate us to get his point across and plenty of times we got hidings. That changed when I was a teenager and became more staunch. Perhaps the testosterone and my size helped put him off.

One day in my early 20s things came to a head. We had a family bank account going and we were all putting in $5 per week. It came to everyone's notice that my brother had ripped a lot of money off to use for gambling. During a family meeting up at the house, things got very heated. In the midst of this Dad started attacking Mum. I immediately got everyone out of the house while Mum and Dad were still arguing in the bedroom. Then I went back in there. Dad was on one side of the bed and Mum was on the other. I said to Mum, 'You go outside; he's not going to do anything.' She walked out behind me, and Dad pushed past me to get at her. As he did so, I grabbed one of his arms firmly, reached over and caught hold of his other arm, then foot-tripped him and landed on top of him. I told him very clearly, 'Mate – you're too old for this shit. It's not happening anymore.' At that point, something shifted. I think he realised he could no longer carry on like that.

Five years prior to that incident, Dad became a born-again Christian. He then pulled away from his gang connections and stopped using drugs. I have been around Christianity most of my life, and I knew it was better for Mum that Dad was changing. However, I believe it took my intervention for him to change his aggressive behaviour towards my mother. I still don't know how I feel about God and spirituality from a religious point of view. My experiences have been Māori-related spiritual incidents rather than Christian ones. I relate more to my Māori side.

My Mum has always had a strong role in my life. She's an extremely hard worker and taught us to take care of everything around the house. She honoured her marriage vows when a lot of people would have walked away. She did her best to protect us. We went to women's refuges quite a few times in the early days. As a mum in those difficult situations, she did an outstanding job.

The year before I met Wiremu, my cousin gave me a book for my birthday. It was about the settlement where my Nan's family have lived for generations. My Nan grew up there with her mother and father in a little shed. Even today there is no power and the folks up there are on creek water. When I read the book, I learnt about the history of that place. Many battles between Māori happened there centuries ago. One of the main chiefs was a ferocious warrior. He was known for his unrelenting fighting ability and the way he avenged the death of close family members. I found myself identifying with this ancestor, with his suffering and his tenacity in the way he approached his battles. He was tactical about everything he did, planning carefully to achieve his goals. And the thing that stood out for me was that he would never give up.

When Wiremu asked me about my ancestor, it was this tipuna that he referred to. The greatest impact from that first meeting with Wiremu was realising I wasn't alone. Even though I had all these people around supporting me, I always felt there was something missing. When Wiremu told me who he could see, I realised that even though I had felt alone, my ancestor had been there all the time.

Reflections on the Nine Years since the Session

In the nine years since I first went to Te Whare Mārie, I have had several occasions when I have become overwhelmed by a bunch of things going wrong all on top of each other. When the depressing thoughts have returned, so have the suicidal thoughts. The last time, about two years ago, things were really getting on top of me. One Friday night I was driving home, and I burst into tears and pulled over in my truck. I'd just had enough. At that point I rang the crisis team. I ended up going to the emergency department. After waiting to see the mental health team, I finally went home without being seen. As suicidal as I was, I knew I wasn't going to act on that.

Since that moment with Wiremu, when I get into the dark holes again and the suicide thoughts return, I think about this chief standing behind me, and tell myself, 'I just need to keep fighting.' But the thing for me is I'm fighting mental battles with myself, in order to keep on going in my life. My most difficult mental battle was with suicide. At my darkest times I felt like I was circling that plughole, going round and round, ready to be sucked down into the vortex of self-destruction and death. Fighting against that, for me, meant going against the current, swimming as hard as I could to get away from it. Back then, it felt quite possible that I could have gone ahead and ended my life. That won't happen now. After that first meeting with Wiremu, I have known that I am protected, even from myself.

I consider that I have only the bare minimum of understanding of my Māori culture as I wasn't brought up involved in it. However, I have always known that I have had some sort of power. Even though I've never really understood it, more recently I relate that power back to my mana. After meeting Wiremu and Tai, I started going back up to our family land almost once a month. I continued that for over six months, and it really felt healing. Up there, I feel very different. I am much calmer. In the city, any noise, such as a car driving past or people talking on the street, will keep me awake. But up on our land the wind may be howling in the trees and the cows mooing all night and I will sleep soundly. Being up there I didn't have to deal with anything; I could just relax and go fishing, walking or hunting. For me I put this sense of calm down to the wairua of the place and the presence of my ancestors. Since that time with Wiremu and Tai, I have become more interested and curious about my heritage. I want to understand it more and find out what my part is in it. I have been encouraging my own kids to learn more about their Māori culture as a result.

I feel privileged to have my ancestor there with me. I wouldn't say I'm always aware of his presence, but I'm confident that he's there in the background as I'm battling along through life. I used to feel self-conscious when I'd talk to myself. But now I know I can talk to my ancestor. Sometimes he seems to wait for things to get hard, so he can step in and help. At other times he's waiting for me to call upon him for assistance. There is a feeling of peace for me that comes through knowing that should the shit hit the fan, I'm protected. As a result, I have more faith in myself. Spiritually, I'm up for whatever life will bring.

Peter

Reflections on the Session

I had been at Te Whare Mārie for three years before the session with Tohu. I came to this service because I always believed that there is a spiritual and a cultural realm. If we can integrate these aspects into how we practice psychiatry, then we have to be adding more value for the people that we see.

In my own background, my father was a Baptist minister, and I always respected his open-mindedness, intelligence and awareness of different viewpoints. I believe the many conversations I had with him sowed seeds in my mind and helped me to be open to a broader range of spiritual perspectives. I don't think it's unusual for us as human beings to have awareness of things beyond the usual dimensions that we exist in. For example, some people might have a certain awareness of a future event. How that works, I don't know. We can't explain it in psychiatry as such, but it happens. The idea that a human being can be aware of something in this room that I can't be aware of is not uncomfortable to me in principle. The uncomfortable part for me in this instance was not having a framework for understanding it.

I was born in the United Kingdom and trained in both medicine and psychiatry there. My psychiatric training was very middle of the road, mainstream psychiatry. Prior to that, while travelling abroad, I worked in mental health in New Zealand for a period with a psychiatrist with a holistic and family-focused outlook, and that encouraged me to return here when I had completed my training. However, there was nothing in any of my medical or psychiatric training to prepare me for this encounter with Wiremu.

Looking back, I have questions around the actual phenomena of what was being observed. At the time, Wiremu's interjection was like a bolt out of the blue. There was no 'I need to say this,' it was just 'Bang!' It gave a sense of, 'Wow, this is huge.' Having assumed I was sitting with a colleague who was an interesting man with strong cultural knowledge, suddenly I was thrown into something completely beyond my imagination and experience. I was thinking, 'Oh my God, what is going on?' And there was no further explanation. Wiremu simply fell silent.

My mind was reeling with questions such as: What have I just experienced? Who is the patient here? What was the process that Wiremu went through? Was this some kind of psychotic revelation for Wiremu? I don't believe he was psychotic at the time, but the problem for me was that we never got to talk about it to help me understand what was going on for him. I can accept it now in a superficial way as some kind of insight, some kind of awareness, some kind of state of consciousness, but I felt frustrated afterwards that we didn't have that dialogue to allow me to understand it more at the time.

As well as his description, it felt like there was a whole other layer of significance which Wiremu understood but which he decided not to share further in the session. It seemed as if there was something else enormous going on. I got a sense from Wiremu that he knew much more than he revealed, as if he had some prior awareness of Tohu or some connections to his family, due to which he felt he needed to attend the session. But that was entirely outside of my awareness and knowledge. And it might be totally erroneous, but it had that feel to it. It wasn't just one of our cultural colleagues coming to support us. From the very beginning it felt like it was way more than that.

Given that Wiremu had implied that all of this should be part of a process that should now go on, I was baffled by the casual nature of Wiremu's suggestion at the end to Tohu that perhaps they might meet up at a later time, with a comment like, 'I'll catch you sometime.' In the face of such a significant event, I felt puzzled that Wiremu would appear so nonchalant.

Despite my bewilderment and questions, the opportunity never arose to have an in-depth conversation with Wiremu about what transpired that day prior to his departure from our service later that year. We did, of course, discuss Tohu at our multidisciplinary meeting and the plans that he would see Wiremu and Tai for some individual cultural therapy. I was pleased that things improved for Tohu quite rapidly, and he was discharged from the service. Nonetheless, at various times since then, I have wondered about what took place. For example, I have reflected on the relevance of what occurred to Tohu's mental health predicament. How could we have worked with what Wiremu saw, in tandem with a New Zealand mainstream model? And most of all, it made me think how useful it would be to have a framework that could encompass both the Māori spiritual side and mainstream Western psychiatric points of view. Would there be some utility in having a crucible that could hold all of this together? These are some of the questions that have lingered with me about that day.

Diagnostic Considerations

On the day of that first meeting, I had a strong sense that Tohu had walked through that door with a lot of depression and anxiety. He had a wide range of symptoms that would have justified a diagnosis of major depression. However, the speed of his improvement, without any conventional psychiatric interventions, led me to conclude that he was suffering from a less severe problem, namely an adjustment disorder as a result of his relationship break-up. Looking back now, I wonder if Wiremu's intervention relieved Tohu's depressive symptoms in a way that I did not appreciate at the time.

Stepping across the Gap

Having read through the perspectives from Tohu, Tai, Wiremu and Allister, I believe I would address such a situation differently in my practice these days. Nine years ago, I had no similar Māori cultural interactions to help me understand it. Now, I would want to step across that doctor-cultural gap and say something like, 'Wow! That blew me away. Please carry on. Please help us understand.' I would want to put the whole psychiatric process to one side and say, 'Look this is important, let's explore this.' I would want to invite Wiremu to open up this space for us and support Tohu coming into that space, in order that we might explore it together.

There are constraints for us as psychiatrists and other professionals in exploring these matters. Some clinicians may hold back, wondering if they will be judged by the system as unprofessional if they talk about spiritual matters. It can take courage to step outside the box; however, at Te Whare Mārie we have an invitation to do that. In order to have an authentic exchange about culture or about spirit with a person meeting me, I believe I need to enter that conversational space mindful of my own culture and spirit. Perhaps that might feel uncomfortable. However, reflection on my own background, culture and spiritual values can give me a stronger base to step outside my own professional and worldviews. That may give me the courage to stretch across that chasm between my beliefs and Māori spiritual values.

Tai

The moment when Wiremu declared that he could see Tohu's ancestor just behind him took me unawares. As he described the physical features of this person, I had the impression he was referring to a distinguished Māori figure like a kaumātua (elder). Of course, I couldn't see anyone there. Shortly after, Tohu confirmed that the figure was likely to be his tipuna. I remember they discussed his name. I was equally amazed that the identity of this person seemed to have so much meaning for Tohu.

While Tohu didn't say much more about it that day, after that initial session, Wiremu and I met with him a number of times. His initial mistrust appeared to be transformed after Wiremu saw his ancestor. Tohu was eager to hear more about what Wiremu had seen that day, and seemed blown away with what Wiremu was able to see and tell him. We talked about the significance of the appearance of this rangatira in his life. Tohu was very warmly engaged on each occasion. Wiremu's knowledge of that ancestor and the area that Tohu's whānau came from mattered a lot to him. Here was someone who could help him make sense of the meaning of these significant matters in his life. Tohu related all this to his background, including his father's gang connections, family violence and the impact of this on his life. After this time, Tohu started going back up to his whānau land up north quite often. He stayed in contact with our service for several months and then felt he was doing much better and no longer needed us.

This was not the only time I have witnessed Wiremu demonstrating his remarkable gift of matekite (spiritual awareness). Sometimes people are surprised to hear me acknowledge this type of gift because they know about my Mormon faith. Perhaps they think that my religion might not allow for such Māori cultural beliefs. However, I grew up with it. My mother and a few of my siblings were also matekite. My mother often had visitations from whānau who were no longer alive whom she called 'people from the other side', especially if there was something wrong that the ancestors wanted to address. She made sure to share these experiences with the rest of us. So Wiremu's abilities were not a surprise to me. There is space in my faith for that kind of thinking. It is my belief that God gives these spiritual gifts to particular people and not just to Mormons. I consider that the purpose of such gifts is to protect, comfort and bless the lives of the recipients and those around them. I have always respected the way Wiremu acknowledges where his gift comes from: from his Source.

Allister

Although I wasn't involved as a psychiatrist with Tohu, when Tai mentioned the incident to me, I wondered if Tohu would consider speaking to me about it. Accordingly, I raised this with Peter and Tai. With Tohu's agreement, our first meeting took place. It was four years after Tohu's first session. I met Tohu with Tai in the reception area at Te Whare Mārie. Tohu was casually dressed in a faded green T-shirt with a trucking logo, black rugby shorts and jandals. Upon standing, he towered over me, greeting me with 'Gidday doc' and a friendly handshake. After we sat down together, even though that time had elapsed, I was struck by the freshness, enthusiasm and immediacy with which Tohu spoke about his experience of meeting Peter, Tai and Wiremu on that first occasion. I noticed his willingness to share his experience with others, in order that they might learn something from it. It was clear to me that he had pondered frequently on the significance of what Wiremu had seen that day, and he talked freely to me about what that meant to him.

It was a further five years later when I sat down with Peter to hear his story. Peter had a warm and friendly style, and dapper appearance. His grey hair was closely cropped, and his professional attire consisted of dark trousers, white shirt and colourful bow tie and braces. I knew that Peter was held in high regard by his Māori colleagues on the pakeke (adult) team and had been unruffled during periods of change and uncertainty for the team.

I was eager to hear Peter's account of the session nine years before. Given the many psychiatric interviews he would have had in the intervening years, I was interested in how vividly he recalled what transpired that day. Clearly that encounter made a deep impression on him, even if it had been hard to fathom. However, one aspect of his story did not surprise me. Peter's bewilderment at Wiremu's revelation about the ancestor in the room and the fact that he had no inkling that Wiremu was capable of perceiving wairua in that way resonated with my own experience of my early work with Wiremu.

When I had an opportunity to hear both Peter's and Wiremu's accounts of the first session with Tohu, it occurred to me that mutual respect had been a factor in the way that session played out. Wiremu's respect for Peter's role and psychiatric protocol explained his reluctance to interrupt and his silence later in the interview. Peter held back from asking Wiremu about his response in deference to Wiremu's cultural authority. Similarly, in regard to Peter's unresolved questions after the interview, I know for myself that with a busy schedule, it would have been easy for weeks and months to pass without Peter managing to approach Wiremu about Tohu and his ancestor. However, there are also socio-historical barriers to communication between a psychiatrist and a Māori healer. As described in Chapter 2, Māori healing was marginalised as a medium of healthcare in Aotearoa and then outlawed by the early 1900s. Psychiatry's dominant role in the hierarchy of mental health services has contributed strongly to the silencing of Māori healing perspectives.

I can also relate to Peter's conundrum about how to make sense of Wiremu's perceptual experience of Tohu's ancestor. In psychiatric training, we are taught to examine the question of whether someone might be having a psychotic experience or not, but we have very little language to describe spiritual experiences that may resemble psychosis. So naturally, because Wiremu had seen someone in the room that Peter couldn't see, it made sense that he was left wondering if Wiremu might be having a hallucination.

Wiremu

Tātaihono

I like Peter's kōrero about the importance of finding a way to make sense of both Western psychiatry views and te ao Māori perspectives. He was advocating for developing ways of working in partnership. During that time, when I first met Tohu, Allister and I were developing our method of collaboration, which I call tātaihono and outlined in Chapter 1. I believe this model provides useful guidance for addressing a number of matters Peter raises.

Wairua or Psychotic Experience?

I am interested in Peter's question about whether it was possible that I was having a psychotic revelation. If I was having a psychotic experience, why would it reveal anything meaningful that could help another person? I would assume that a psychotic experience could be disturbing and is unlikely to be useful for a healing purpose. Because I have experiences like this so frequently, I am often seeking to make sense of them. I am happy to consider many types of explanations and open to suggestions. Sometimes I even question myself about whether I am having psychotic experiences. However, because I am often able to discover a reason for my experiences of hearing, seeing and knowing things that are not apparent to others, I am generally confident that they are wairua experiences. In addition, in the last 30 or 40 years I have been able to use these experiences to guide my healing work, and other people find this helpful. As a result, I have concluded that the things I see and hear represent matekite experiences and that they are provided to me for a healing purpose.

My kuia taught me that every wairua experience was meaningful and it was all part and parcel of who we were. She taught me that there was always a reason, and it was not a coincidence that I had been given an experience. She told me that these things had been given in order that I might help someone, that these experiences had to be treated carefully, and that people had to be treated with respect.

During this experience, I saw someone, I got an immediate feeling about the mana of this rangatira, and shortly after this I realised who this renowned ancestor was. There were several ways I perceived him. This is more than just purely seeing, which is what the term 'visual hallucination' implies to me. The holistic unity of my experience tells me this comes from wairua. With regards to a message, while Tohu's tipuna didn't have a simple communication for me to relay to him verbally, this presence carried a very powerful implicit message: that his ancestor was here with him. In addition, Tohu's sudden realisation of the direct link with his ancestor and his whakapapa made a huge impact on him. This was not a random hallucination. This relationship between my experience and Tohu's situation is characteristic of wairua.

When I consider the outcome, Tohu said he was much less likely to act on his suicidal thoughts following our hui. He felt more connected to his whenua and whānau, and curious about his whakapapa and Māori culture. His wellbeing improved. He was more confident to tackle the problems in his life. So it appears that the fruits of the experience I had were positive and, I would say, healing for Tohu. In contrast, psychotic symptoms such as hallucinations are defined by the negative effects that they have on people. Someone wouldn't be labelled with a psychotic illness unless the results were quite negative on their life.

Healing

Although I do healing work, I don't consider myself to be the healer. I believe that seeing, hearing and knowing are provided by my Source. Any information I may offer gives that person an opportunity to heal themselves.

This healing could be through spiritual changes they make in their lives, their belief in their ability to have authority over their circumstances, or relational changes they might make following that interaction.

For Tohu, healing seemed to come about through hearing about the presence of his ancestor and realising the significance of his connection to this chiefly line in his whakapapa. Suddenly he was faced with the knowledge that he was not alone.

There is a saying: 'Ehara taku mana, i te mana takitahi, engari he mana takimano' (My mana is not just mine alone. It belongs to a multitude of my people.).

I believe knowing of the presence of his ancestor allowed Tohu to have a totally new perspective on his mana, identity and life circumstances.

7 Grace

Wiremu NiaNia, Hazel, Allister Bush, and David Epston

Grace was 11 when she started hearing voices and seeing visions. She heard a man's voice telling her to harm herself and had repeated visions of a man watching her. A few months earlier, she'd watched as her father assaulted her mother, after which she began suffering from flashbacks, nightmares and disturbed sleep.

This chapter tells the story of a family healing session involving Grace, her mother, Hazel, her two siblings, her grandmother Mele and family pastor, Paula, with Wiremu and Allister. During the session Grace's courageous action to banish this apparition is revealed, coinciding with the resolution of her voices and visions. This outcome illustrates an important principle in Wiremu's Māori healing approach: restoration of spiritual authority is pivotal in protecting those affected by spiritual problems. In addition, Wiremu highlights the necessity of addressing unresolved relational distress to restore the collective spiritual authority of the family and further protect Grace's wellbeing. He supports Grace's Samoan, Tokelau and Cook Island family in their Christian faith while at the same time encouraging them to consider the significance of family violence as a relational breach which is important to address.

Following this account of the session, the next sections provide reflections from Allister, Wiremu and Hazel. Allister considers possible causes for Grace's experiences and describes the follow-up session with Grace and her family. Next, Wiremu explains his analysis of Grace's voices and visions, why he concluded that Grace was suffering from a spiritual problem, the strong steps the family had already taken to address this predicament and wairua (spiritual) approaches to address a relational breach. Finally, 18 months and then five years after the session, Hazel reflects on Grace's progress and the impact of this collaborative healing process on the whole family.

DOI: 10.4324/9781003187042-7

Allister

Grace's Family Healing Session

'I was trying to figure out where the sound of crying was coming from,' Hazel began.

It was all dark in the house, and I was listening. I wondered if I was imagining it. A little while later Grace's sister Nadia called out from her room, 'I can hear someone calling out "Help me."' At first, I thought she was mistaken. Perhaps she had overheard some people outside on our street. Not long after, there was a thud and a crash, and I heard Grace jump out of bed and stomp her way to the kitchen. I could hear her pour herself a glass of water.

When she made her way back to bed, past my room, I could see that she had been crying. I called out to her, 'What's up, love?' At first, she tried to pretend she was okay, but then she just sat on the end of my bed and started sobbing. She wouldn't look at me. Finally, she burst out, 'I can hear this voice. It's a man's voice. It won't leave me alone. It told me when I die it has the funeral planned for me. It has the casket and pillow all ready. It said that I'm not allowed to tell you because you won't believe me.'

I put my arms around her and told her, 'I do believe you!' At that moment she looked at me and I could see the relief on her face.

Hazel turned to look at Grace, who was sitting next to her in our fono (meeting) room at Health Pasifika. Grace nodded and met her gaze, and Hazel reached out to put her hand on Grace's knee. Wiremu and I were listening intently to Hazel's story, along with Mele, Hazel's mother; Paula; and Grace's sister Nadia, aged eight, who was on the floor playing with their baby sister.

'So that was the first night,' said Hazel.

> The next night it happened again. This time, Grace was in the shower. The girls had been having a singing battle, so the house was quite noisy. All of a sudden, Grace went quiet. After a few moments she came sprinting out of the bathroom, wrapped in her towel and in tears. I said, 'Babe, what's the matter?' She responded, 'I heard that voice again. It told me to use the shower hose to hang myself.' I felt shocked. I sat her down, held her and prayed for her. By this time, we were both crying.'

Even though I'd heard Hazel's story when we had our first assessment meeting eight weeks earlier, I still felt moved by it. We'd invited Grace to tell some of the story, but she'd said she preferred her mother to speak about it. Wiremu, who was meeting the family for the first time, urged Hazel to continue.

After that, Grace stayed in my room for a few nights. That weekend she attended a church camp. Two nights after her return she was in her room and heard the voice once more. This time all it said was, 'Hi Grace.' She freaked out again and came back into my room. The following night Grace let me know that the voice had greeted her the same way, this time when she was in the toilet. Again, I had her sleep in with me and we were all praying for her. By this time, I had made an appointment with our family doctor. She referred us to Health Pasifika.

Over the following couple of weeks, I was concerned about Grace. She wasn't herself. She would go into little trances. She was more argumentative with her sister and me. Nadia was upset with me for not telling Grace off like I normally would when she was naughty. One time, Nadia said she had seen something strange about Grace's eyes when she looked at her, telling me her eyes were just 'black as ever'. I told her, 'I know, baby. That's why I can't growl at her because I don't think it's her.'

Every night I always see my kids to bed and kiss them goodnight. Then I clean the house up, shower, and go back and kiss them again once they are asleep. During that time, whenever I would return to Grace's room, I felt like something was there. Something was in her room, looking at me, not wanting me to go in there by her. It didn't feel good. I would just walk into her room like, 'Hell no, this is my house, that is my baby!' I would go in there and I would pray for her.

During this time, I spoke a lot with our pastor, Paula. One weekend she arranged for some elders from our church to come round to our house. We had a prayer meeting that lasted a couple of hours. After that the voice didn't come back for a while. Grace seemed a bit better in herself. I thought, 'Okay, we are slowly getting our girl back.'

It was a week or two later, after our first appointment here at Health Pasifika, that the next thing happened. Grace had been off school during some of this time, and when she returned, I explained to her teacher what had been happening. One day her teacher phoned me. 'Grace had a bit of an incident today. After lunch she had been to the toilet and on her return, I could see that she was visibly shaken so I had taken her to one side and asked her what was wrong. She said that while she was in the toilet she heard the voice again, just saying, "Hello Grace."'

Wiremu interrupted to ask if the voice was male or female, and Hazel clarified that it was male.

> Within a few nights, something changed. I was doing some baking in the kitchen. Grace got up out of bed to go to the toilet and shortly after she rushed out and came running to me in tears and exclaimed, 'Mum, it's a

man! He's standing there in the bathroom.' I went to have a look. There was nothing I could see, but now I was thinking, okay, I think I know what this is. It was looking more and more like a spiritual problem. I was feeling increasingly angry about this intrusive stubborn thing harassing my daughter. Several moments later she screamed again, 'Mum, he's standing there by the Christmas tree!' Again, I was holding her and praying for her.

During this time, I was thinking a lot about what Grace told me about her experience. She said the voice sounded husky, like a smoker's voice. But she wasn't sure if the voice was connected to the man she saw because his face didn't look like he was speaking. She told me the man she saw had a dark complexion, spiky black hair and was wearing a black mask. His eyes and mouth looked red. After this incident, my father suggested I get in touch with our landlord, to find out what had gone on previously in the house.

At that point Hazel asked Grace if she and her sisters could go into the reception area, as she wanted to talk about some adult matters. Once they'd departed, Hazel continued talking.

The following night Grace was off to have a shower, and I asked her if she would like me to sit in there with her, and she said yes. Her baby sister was running up and down the hallway in her walker, pulling all the dirty clothes out of the laundry basket. Just as I stepped out of the bathroom to intervene, Grace screamed: 'Aaagh! He's here again!' When I got back in there, she was trying to cover herself up with the shower curtain. 'Honest to God, Mum, he's standing there staring at me! Shall I talk to him? Shall I ask him what he wants?' My response was, 'No, no you don't need to talk to it.' I said, 'Come on!' I turned the shower off, wrapped Grace in a towel and we went out to the living room.

I called our landlord half an hour later. I began, 'I don't know how to approach this without offending you in any way. But there have been a few things going on with my daughter and now she has been seeing something in this house. Is there anything that may have happened in this house in the past that you think I should know about?' He said, 'Do you mean like a murder?' I responded, 'Well, anything at all.' He went on, 'There's not really much I can think of. Originally this was a poor man's house. After my parents bought it, we grew up here but nothing really bad happened. There was this one time when my parents were concerned that something bad had followed us home. But our church minister came and prayed for the house, and everything seemed fine after that.'

It was then that he offered to come round and pray for us. My first thought was, 'Oh, that would be good.' However, shortly after he knocked on the door and I invited him in, I began to feel really uncomfortable. It was a quarter to nine at night, and being a single lady, alone at home with my children, there was something about his manner that made me feel very uneasy. Anyway, he strode confidently into our house and had all these pretty words to say but the entire time he was speaking I was feeling very intimidated. I just sat there with my head bowed. I didn't trust what he was doing. Meanwhile, he was saying, 'Between the three of us, you [speaking to Grace] have the authority over your body, and your Mum, she is the authority of your household, and me, I have authority over this house.' No, you do not, I thought. This is getting more weird. Next, he said, 'I am going to pray,' and he started without waiting for my response.

As he began, my spirit was feeling very unsettled. I couldn't look at him. I couldn't even tell him, 'Please don't pray! I don't know what that prayer is, and I do not know where you are drawing your power or energy from!' He just kept praying love and light and had this really over-the-top charm thing going on. Nadia was saying, 'Go on, mum. If he is praying to God, this is good!' I looked at her, and in my mind, I was thinking, no it's not! And Nadia gave me a strange look. Meanwhile, my landlord was walking through praying over the house. I couldn't pray; I couldn't even think clearly. He returned in a few moments and invited Grace to come for a walk around the house and pray with him. Before I could intervene, she said okay. I followed them, feeling even more agitated. I heard Grace telling him, 'I do not like the bathroom, I can't go in there.' Immediately he walked right in there, turned on the light and started praying again. He then turned to Grace and asked, 'Would you like to say anything?' To my surprise she spoke up. 'Yes. Yes, I would!' Stepping into the bathroom, she closed her eyes and spoke in the most courageous, powerful voice I have ever heard from her. 'In the name of Jesus, get out! With all my heart, in Jesus' name, I demand that you leave!' What she said snapped me out of whatever I was feeling. Suddenly I could speak again. I sat there and agreed with her. 'Yes Lord, you have authority over my house; you are the centre of my house.' As soon as he had finished praying, I ushered him out of the house immediately. I locked the door and straightaway I burst out crying. I didn't trust what he had done in our house. Once I had some time to calm myself, I led the girls around the house, and we prayed for each room; we asked for Jesus' protection over every wall he had touched. I was so shaken that there and then I decided we were going to my Mum and Dad's place. The same night we packed up our things, closed up the house and drove to their place.

> We returned to our house a few weeks later. Since that night, Grace has not seen or heard anything untoward. She still asks me to come and sit in the bathroom while she has a shower, but she is starting to get more confident with that.

At this point I interrupted Hazel to ask if we could bring the girls back into the room. 'I would like Grace to hear your story about her telling this thing to get lost. I think it is quite a powerful story.'

After they had returned and Hazel had repeated the story, Wiremu spoke up. 'In order for us to make sense of what is happening for Grace, I often talk about a process of elimination to help determine what is going on,' he explained.

> As Christians, we have a tendency to assume that everything that we don't understand is demonic. And sometimes our worldviews as Indigenous people, for me as Māori, and for you as Samoan, Tokelau and Cook Island, have been stigmatised as part of that. In my work I deal with the spirit. There is a saying in Māori, 'I hangaia tātou ki te Atua, te hīkoi tātou, te hīkoi tāngata,' which means that first and foremost we are spiritual beings experiencing a human existence. I look to the spiritual side first. And you have all looked after that side. There is enough faith here to move a maunga (mountain) to the other side of town. With all the prayers at your home, with your pastor and in your church, you have taken care of that. So, I am thinking, what's going on that helps this thing, this gremlin, to keep coming back?
>
> 'Now, before our session, I asked Allister not to tell me any details about your situation. I prefer to meet you all fresh and see what comes up.' Wiremu turned to me. 'But before our session, I did mention to you that there is something about a man in the shower. Do you remember that, Allister?'

I nodded, and he continued. 'So, I already had an idea you were dealing with something like this. We often talk about looking at the spiritual side, the physical side, the mental side and the relational side. All these aspects are important. And while I might leave the physical side to the doctors, I am interested in the spiritual side, but I also want to consider other aspects.'

Mele emphasised that she had advised Hazel to ring her doctor. 'It's important to have the medical and psychological sides looked at, even while we eliminate some of the spiritual side.'

Wiremu agreed. 'Alongside those other aspects, let's consider the relational side, for example. When I talk about the relational side, I am talking about relationships with our ancestors, or our immediate whānau (family) dynamics. But I also include our relationships to our environment and the places where we stay. Sometimes unresolved conflict in the lives of our forefathers and mothers can come down upon the younger ones. Other times the key lies in relationships in this generation. Maybe we need to check ourselves as a family. Is there something there that we need to address before that prayer is answered? Because for me God is mighty, but something is still holding back the full power of that prayer. Does that make sense? Sometimes someone has had their mana (spiritual authority) trodden on, or been hurt or belittled in front of others. And they may have felt really stink and there has been no opportunity for reparation, for that mana to be restored.'

'I hear what you are saying,' said Mele. She looked at Hazel, 'There is another thing. Are you okay if I talk about that?' Hazel met her gaze and nodded. Mele took a slow breath and continued. 'Grace's parents had a pretty bad break-up. Just before they broke up, one night the girls witnessed their Dad beating up their mother very badly. There had been heated arguments before, but that was the first time they had seen anything like that. I know Grace was deeply affected by this. They all were.'

I hadn't briefed Wiremu on this assault before the session, but it had been a focus in our initial child psychiatry family assessment meeting. Grace had difficulties sleeping and had nightmares about the assault, which had happened nine months earlier. Anything that reminded her of the assault would trigger vivid and frightening memories, which would leave her feeling very shaken up. She had refused to see her father since and had been struggling to focus at school; everyone agreed she wasn't herself. In our initial meeting, I'd concluded Grace had enough symptoms to justify a diagnosis of post-traumatic stress disorder and had explained some possible approaches. I decided to raise these approaches again with Grace.

'When we last met, Grace, you were having flashbacks, as you called them, relating to that day when your Dad hurt your Mum,' I said. 'One approach I talked about that could help resolve that traumatic experience was the eye movement therapy called EMDR [Eye Movement Desensitisation Reprocessing]. That would be addressing the trauma from the psychological side. However, Wiremu, I think you are suggesting some kind of spiritual way of addressing the impact of this trauma on the family. Am I right?'

'Yes,' replied Wiremu.

> Another part of my mahi (work) involves working with Māori whānau when there has been family violence. I always ensure that men I'm working with understand that from a Māori point of view, women are a most precious taonga (something treasured) for our whānau, and need to be treated with utmost respect. I can't speak for Samoan,

Tokelau or Cook Island cultures, but in te ao Māori (the Māori world), women are sometimes referred to as the whare tangata. Whare tangata literally means "the house of people." It is out of women that our offspring grow.

Alongside this, it follows that if we give respect to each other, then each person's space is sacred. So, I have to respect that space. Where there has been violence, then that constitutes a breach of that relationship. Such a violation could render someone in the whānau vulnerable to a negative spiritual thing like this. When that happens, it can be helpful to address this relational breach spiritually.

There are a number of ways we can do that. Sometimes it is appropriate to bring everyone into the room together to address what happened. But maybe it's not safe to do that straightaway. When the tāne (man) isn't ready to take responsibility for that violence, that relational breach, then we often need to find other means to seek resolution in the wairua. One way is a process of releasing past hurts that I refer to as whakawetewete. This process doesn't need everyone in the same room. Those who are ready can write down all the painful things, all the things that have hurt you, as well as anything you have done to hurt someone else; everything you want to let go of. Take as much time as you need. Then when you have finished, seal it all up in an envelope, and together you can go down to the beach or wherever you like and make a hole in the sand for all your envelopes. Then you can say a prayer and set fire to the envelopes, handing the contents over to God and your ancestors. No one else ever needs to read what you put in there. Once this is done, it is not your burden to carry any more.

The discussion then focused on several questions the family had about this process.

I (Allister) was still pondering the significance of the moment in the bathroom when Grace had commanded the thing she saw to leave. When I raised this, Hazel spoke up, 'It's interesting that it hasn't come back since then, has it? You stamped your mark and said, "Get out of here! This is our home; me, my Mum and my sister's home."'

Wiremu responded,

I'm not surprised it hasn't shown its face. When you did that, you took your authority back. You took charge. And there was something else you did when you told that thing to get lost. You said, "In the name of Jesus". Through our relationship with God, we are given this ability to have authority over anything that is impinging on our space. That includes anything that might be harassing you in a spiritual way.

Wiremu then explained how Grace seeing her Dad hurting her Mum was important. When something like that happens, it's like a gap in the spiritual protection you get from your family can open up just enough for this thing to try to scare you with that voice and the man you saw. That negative spiritual thing was trying to take advantage. However, you can address this by taking charge of your space, like you did, and for the adults to make sure what happened between your Dad and your Mum gets resolved safely.

Wiremu's comment reminded Hazel that Grace had spent a couple of days in hospital with an infection the previous week. While she was there, Grace told Hazel she wanted to see her Dad.

'She was worried I wouldn't be OK about that,' said Hazel.

> I said to her, 'It is not about me; if you want your Dad to visit, he can.' Grace hadn't seen him for nine months after the assault, and during that period he had spent time in jail. Grace and her sister had been very much on my side at that time. Out of loyalty to me, I think they hadn't allowed themselves to express their feeling of missing their Dad. So, I rang him, and he came into the hospital for a couple of hours. I could see she was so excited to see him. Even though I am still quite wary around him, during that visit he and I had an opportunity to speak together when we left the ward to get a coffee. That was our first conversation in many months. I was able to explain to him about the experiences that Grace had been having, and he was quite concerned. He told me for the first time about some of his own spiritual experiences growing up in Samoa.
>
> After that, the girls asked if they might see him again. Following Grace's discharge from hospital, I agreed they could visit him at his parents' place. That was last Monday night. Since then, I notice Grace looks happier, as if some weight has been lifted from her. It feels like some kind of breakthrough. Even though I still don't trust him due to what happened, I believe that he loves our girls and would want to do the right thing to support them.

As we were nearing the end of the session, I asked Wiremu if he thought there was a spiritual matter he needed to address; whether there was anything negative still hanging on.

'Until these things are addressed, it will still be hanging around,' said Wiremu.

> We know God will free her, there is nothing that can withstand that, but I think there has still been something lurking and the reason is that we need to look at the unresolved relational matters. And you, Grace, and your family have begun to address that.

I encouraged the family to consider Wiremu's explanation and how this might apply in their lives. Wiremu said the whānau had done all the work, and his role was to offer some facilitation. He acknowledged the significant role the pastor had played, and light-heartedly said he'd felt slightly intimidated by her presence.

Everyone laughed, and Paula replied, 'Please don't be intimidated! You are far more experienced than I am, and so I'm keen to be guided by you. I'm just wanting to confirm: in your spirit, is it saying it is safe for me to take my spiritual authority and do what the family are wanting done, like we have been?'

Wiremu agreed it was safe for Paula to continue to pray for the family and for everyone to continue with their spiritual practices. Despite the initial cautious atmosphere, by this stage there was an easy and energetic exchange of stories and ideas, punctuated by moments of boisterous laughter. Humour could be helpful, said Wiremu; it could remind any negative spiritual entities hanging around that they were of no significance.

Hazel reflected on the journey the family had been on since they joined Paula's church. 'When Grace was little, we never used to go to church, and I hadn't talked to her or Nadia about Jesus. However, around the time she was four years old, she asked to go to Sunday school. I was taken aback by that and asked her why. She said her friends went and they said it was cool. Because we knew a few people in this church, a friend offered to take the girls, and with some initial mixed feelings I ended up going along too. After that my Mum came too. So, through Grace wanting to go, my entire family started coming to church.'

I observed that Grace seemed to have been a leader for the family even at that early age. Hazel and Mele nodded in agreement, and Wiremu said, 'Well, at least she had a better answer than my girl. When I asked my girl why she wanted to go to Sunday school, she told me it was because they have good biscuits.' Everyone laughed.

I knew Hazel had wondered whether to invite Wiremu to bless their home, but when I mentioned it Wiremu said he didn't think it would be necessary. 'Nah, I'm confident that you all have this handled well.'

Before the Session with Wiremu

Prior to the family session with Wiremu, I had been thinking about how to understand the voice Grace talked about and the visions she had of a male figure that were so disturbing for her. I considered several potential explanations and diagnoses, and noted the possible relationship between Grace's traumatic experiences and the voice she heard. It is common for people with post-traumatic experiences to have frightening recollections of a voice or an image associated with the traumatic event, often of such an intensity that voices or visions may be experienced as 'real' at that moment. I wondered if her auditory and visual experiences were caused by a traumatic brain process in which she might be stuck in 'trauma time', where the memory appears to be happening right now. This hypothesis, which was discussed in Chapter 4, could be consistent with the threatening content in what the voice had to say and its references to death.

Grace's description of the voice and the male figure appearing to her in the shower were also consistent with auditory and visual hallucinations that could represent a psychotic illness. However, she was young to be experiencing her first psychotic episode and had no other psychotic symptoms, such as delusional beliefs or disorganised thoughts. Severe depression can be associated with negative voices and visions, but, despite Grace's distress at times, she didn't have sustained depressed mood in the weeks leading up to our first meeting. As described in Chapter 4, hallucinatory experiences could also be caused by organic brain problems, such as seizures, or other physical health problems, such as infections or inflammatory conditions in the brain. But the family doctor who had referred Grace to our service had examined her physically and carried out some simple investigations, and hadn't identified a physical health problem.

After Grace's emphatic dismissal of the male figure in the bathroom on the night of the landlord's visit, she had no further experiences of hearing the male voice or seeing the male figure. However, she remained anxious, and at the time of our initial meeting continued to have occasional flashbacks of the assault on her mother. Hallucinations caused by seizures or psychotic disorders don't typically resolve abruptly in the wake of such assertive action. If the voice and visions of the male figure were post-traumatic symptoms, I wasn't clear how their sudden cessation might be explained in this timeframe, given that she was still having the flashbacks.

Our initial agreed treatment plan focused on addressing Grace's ongoing post-traumatic stress symptoms and the impact of the traumatic events on all the family. I suggested to Grace and Hazel that Grace's traumatic memories could be addressed with EMDR therapy, alongside sessions with the family. The theory of EMDR is that traumatic memories can become stuck in an unprocessed form, easily triggered by traumatic reminders. Grace was open to trying EMDR, and Hazel said she would talk these ideas over with her mother and other close friends and family. However, I was aware that the family had strong spiritual values and that their faith and relationship with their church was central in their lives. Over the past decade, I'd also sat in on Wiremu's sessions with Māori young people and their families and seen instances where he'd been able to successfully address a disturbing problem that looked psychiatric but that he believed had its genesis in an unresolved spiritual problem (Bush & NiaNia, 2012; NiaNia et al., 2013; NiaNia et al. 2017a, 2017b). I'd met Pacific young people in the past – including Caleb, from Chapter 1 – who were having vivid perceptual experiences that family members, Wiremu and other people had confidently referred to as spiritual experiences. I was intrigued that the timing of the cessation of Grace's voices and visions fitted well with a Māori healing explanation I had heard Wiremu give many times about the critical role of spiritual authority in protecting a young person and their family from negative spiritual entities.

After seeking advice from my Samoan colleagues, I talked to Grace's family about whether they were interested in consulting with Wiremu. At Health Pasifika, it would be usual practice to suggest that families consult with healers from their own culture. However, at that time, the family didn't have a close association with such a healer, and nor did we as a service. I told Hazel about my experience of working with Wiremu and gave Hazel an article to read about his work with a Cook Island family (NiaNia et al., 2013). I had reservations about arranging for the family to see a New Zealand Māori healer, due to their Samoan, Tokelau and Cook Island heritage, and spoke to Hazel about my misgivings about the possible cultural mismatch. After talking to her mother and pastor, she decided she would like a session with Wiremu.

While writing this chapter, I listened again to the audiotape of the session with Wiremu and Grace's aiga (family). In attempting to put together a coherent narrative that is comprehensible for readers, it is easy for the energy and chaotic feel of a live family session to be sanitised out of the retelling. During that session, there were noisy interactions between siblings going on in the background. Later in the meeting, adults chimed in on top of each other with their own responses to Wiremu's ideas.

Follow-up with Grace and Her Family after the Session

When we met up for our next appointment a month after the session with Wiremu, Hazel introduced me to Grace's father, Mika. Despite their separation, Hazel had asked him to attend our appointment so he could gain a better understanding of Grace's situation and hear about what we'd discussed during the family session with Wiremu. I noticed that Grace was looking relaxed and happy in her parents' presence.

Grace reported no further experiences of hearing a voice or seeing the male figure. She'd had no further flashbacks about the assault, and no nightmares. She and her mother and sisters had all been back in the family home for a few weeks. Grace was still keen for her mother to be nearby when she was in the shower and liked to have the light on in the hallway outside her bedroom at night. I asked her what she thought about meeting Wiremu. 'I liked him,' she told me. 'He didn't judge what I was going through. It was nice to meet him.'

When I spoke with Hazel a few weeks later, she identified two moments that had made the most impact on her during the session with Wiremu. The first was when Wiremu said to me, 'Didn't I ask you about a man in the shower?' She explained, 'In response, you looked at him as if to say, yeah, you did, and he said, "Oh okay, never mind." That really surprised me. It felt good being there with somebody who looks at the spiritual side of things.'

The second moment related to Wiremu's comment about her relationship with Mika. 'That was an important moment for me,' said Hazel. 'He said, you can have the most powerful prayers ever, but if the relationships are not going right, there could still be a problem. That made a lot of sense to me. As a result of that I realised that I needed to address some unresolved matters with my ex-partner, for the sake of the girls.'

Over the following months Grace remained well and happy. When I spoke with her and her mother about the trauma therapy we had previously discussed, she reassured me that, as she was feeling fine, it was no longer required. Some months later we all agreed that she be discharged from our service.

In the meantime, I had talked with Hazel about the possibility of writing about Grace's story. After speaking to Grace and the family, Hazel responded enthusiastically to this proposal. When I contacted Hazel 18 months after the session with Wiremu to ask for her reflections, I was pleased to hear that Grace had had no further experiences of the voice or visions or any other symptoms of concern.

Wiremu

Reflections on the Family Healing Session

Even before meeting Grace, I was confident that there was a spiritual problem impinging on her wellbeing. Before the session, I had seen and felt in the wairua that there was a man in the shower. Once our session was under way, although I didn't want to scare Grace, I was aware of something that felt and looked dark lurking near her. It was a darkness that made me think of something that hadn't been addressed, like anger or violence. I can't say it had a shape: it was just there. I could detect it behind her and around her. Sometimes I liken these things to being in a room where someone has farted half an hour an hour before, and the odour has mostly dissipated, but you can still detect a whiff of it.

However, during our session it became clear to me that Grace and her whānau had already taken significant steps to address this. I liked how Hazel had taken Grace's experiences seriously. She was trying to understand what her daughter was telling her. Together the whānau recognised that she might have a spiritual problem and they were addressing that by means of their faith and prayers. They sought guidance from their pastor and other elders in their church. They are a close-knit whānau and they were turning to each other for support.

I noticed that they weren't panicking about whether she might have a mental health problem like psychosis. However, they still sought advice from their doctor and came in to see Allister at Health Pasifika.

Most reassuring to me was Grace's approach. When Grace took the bull by the horns, stepped into the bathroom and told that thing to get lost, the voice and visions that she had before ceased. At that moment she connected with her Source and took her own authority back. That told me that she could stand her ground and wouldn't let this thing push her around anymore. From then on it had less power over her; its influence was diminishing. After hearing that she could take that authority, I knew that this would help her to spiritually ward off any unseen negative influences.

When we met, the whānau were open to what I had to say. While they might have had some reservations about meeting with a Māori healer, they did it anyway. I think they were determined to find a solution. During our session, they listened to the kōrero, and they were able to expand their thinking. In particular, they were open to reflecting on the significance of relational problems in their family life.

There are some whānau that I would karakia (pray) for. However, in this case, I didn't need to. I was satisfied that they could sort it out. Even though the spiritual problem was still lurking, they understood that what was required was to address the relational problem. They needed to put a nail in that box and finish it off. It's not always helpful for a whānau to become dependent on me to karakia for them. I prefer to give the authority back to them and so I invited their pastor to finish our session with a prayer. My role is to tautoko (support) their process. I would rather do myself out of a job.

There is a saying, 'Ko te tangata e tohu ana ki te marama, ehara ko ia te marama,' which means, the person who points to the moon is not the moon. Even though I might be able to provide guidance, I believe healing comes from Te Kaihanga (The Creator). I will do whatever I can to encourage them to connect to that Source. I felt that they were already on to that. It was interesting for me that the family brought their pastor along to the session. Obviously, Grace and Hazel come from a Christian family, and I wonder if they wanted to make sure that there wasn't any conflict between the Christian side and the cultural side. I would say that it is fair dinkum for them to be wondering where I am coming from spiritually. I try not to impose what I believe on people. I just go with where their religious beliefs and values are up to, unless I have some concern that a particular belief is problematic. If that is the case, I will find a way to address it. I don't mind what religious tradition people adhere to. Whatever their beliefs I will treat them the same way: with respect.

When Hazel told the story of the landlord coming to the house, it was clear that he didn't ask for permission to start praying for them. Consent is very important in any wairua work. In my mahi, I am very careful to always seek agreement from the whānau before proceeding with spiritual work. If I am in any doubt about that, I won't proceed. In the wairua practitioner certification courses my wife, Lesley, and I run, to train more spiritual practitioners who can interface with clinical services, seeking permission is a fundamental ethical practice that we frequently remind our students about. As a result of not seeking permission, the landlord breached a relational boundary and was treading on the spiritual authority of the family. That house was their space. They had authority over it, even though he was the landlord. He invaded their space, and so I believe that Hazel was right to be concerned about his actions.

Grace's story provides an example of a young person who was hearing a voice and seeing a vision that others such as her mother couldn't see. Very often, talking about experiences like this will lead to a young person coming to the attention of a mental health service or clinician. Without guidance from a wairua practitioner or kaumātua (elder), it may be difficult for clinicians to help a young person make sense of wairua experiences or even recognise them in the first place. When I met Grace, I already sensed that there was a negative spiritual entity affecting her. However, for those who don't have that intuition, it can be hard to recognise.

The details of what Grace described about her experience can help us clarify the possible origin of this problem. When I heard her description, I was thinking about a wairua problem, and usually I can detect something in the wairua to explain those experiences. However, another clinician might be wondering about other problems such as trauma or psychosis or perhaps that her imagination was running wild.

The message that was coming through from this voice was that she would have to succumb to the voice's command and direction. It was telling her, 'I'm the boss.' The voice was manipulating her in order to gain control and persuade her that she was helpless. It sounded to me like it was playing into the bad experience that she'd had. The traumatic experience made her more psychologically vulnerable to this entity, as she could be easily triggered into fearing that she was going crazy or that something bad was going to happen. When I thought about the connection between Grace and this thing, I was considering possible links with past or current events in her life. Because of the negative nature of this presence, I was wondering about unresolved family conflict or events going back in her family line. By the end of the session, I was confident her experience of the voice was connected to that traumatic incident.

With regard to the fruits of this presence, they can be judged from its impact on Grace's wellbeing: she's experiencing distress, she's fearful, she's not able to focus at school. This thing tells her she will die and not to talk to her mother. That suggests to me a malevolent influence. I've often noticed that negative entities afflict young people with the most potential to benefit others in the whānau, perhaps with an intention to stunt the growth of that capacity.

At the same time, it's interesting to reflect on the big picture. We can accept that this presence had negative intent, but I prefer to step back from labelling these things as all good or all bad. Even if an apple is rotten, it can still make good compost. Due to this wairua problem, Grace has learnt a lot about herself. She has discovered that she had the spiritual authority to take charge of her space and banish this thing. All whānau members have learnt more about wairua alongside their Christian views. Ultimately, they have been addressing unresolved hurts that could have gone unattended for many years. The pastor was also open to learning something new about wairua. I consider myself a student of what others teach me, and Grace's situation is no exception. Furthermore, in giving permission for this story to be shared with you, our reader, the whānau have ensured that a lot more good can come out of this scenario.

At the time, I had concerns for Grace's father. Even though he wasn't present, I still felt he would need help. His act or acts of violence would have come from somewhere. There is a question in te reo Māori (the Māori language), 'He aha te pūtake?' which refers to looking for the root cause. I was sure that the origin of that violence lay in his own experiences earlier in his life. If I could have met him, I would have been interested to explore this further and see if I could assist him to address that. Jail doesn't fix the problem. Jail just punishes you for the act. If we are walking in wairua, we are protected. If we obey the tikanga (protocol) of respecting someone's mana, we are protected. If I breach a tapu, then I no longer have that protection, and if I am the mother or father in the family then the consequences of that can affect my children. The korowai, the protection that is afforded them from the mana of the whole family, may be compromised and can make them susceptible to negative influences. I was happy to read Hazel's account below and to hear that Grace's father has been able to have some healing for his own mamae (hurt) over the last several years.

Hazel

18 Months after the Family Healing Session

When I look back, I felt quite anxious about meeting Wiremu in the days leading up to our session with him. I wasn't sure what to expect, especially after the experience with my landlord. I was also influenced by scary ghost stories about people meeting with tohunga (Māori healers) or Pacific healers. I had never imagined we would be part of that. At the same time, Allister had shown me a photo of Wiremu the week before we met him, and he looked friendly. I decided I wouldn't open up if I didn't feel comfortable. I would wait and see. I didn't know if I would be able to trust him or the process or not. And I wasn't at all ready to tell our story again.

Soon after Wiremu walked into the room, I began to feel comfortable with him. Even though I had never met him before, I can remember noticing that warm fuzzy feeling that you feel when you meet a good friend that you haven't seen for a while. I felt unexpectedly peaceful. He had a friendly expression on his face. He seemed honest and genuine to me. When he spoke during our round of introductions, what he said made me feel at ease and after that I felt okay about telling the story.

Our family has Samoan, Tokelau and Cook Island sides. Even though I identify with my Samoan side, during my growing up here in New Zealand, I have had a lot to do with New Zealand Māori culture. While sometimes there can be a rivalry between our cultures, I usually feel quite comfortable being around Māori friends and situations. All of my kids love Māori culture and love te reo. So even though Wiremu is Māori, meeting him felt quite natural for me.

Another thing that worried me beforehand was about his religious beliefs. It mattered to me whether he believed in Jesus or not. I'm a born-again Christian, but I don't know many Māori who are born-again. Many Māori that I know belong to the Rātana Church or are Mormon. I felt anxious because I just wasn't sure that this man would take my beliefs seriously. After meeting him, I still wasn't sure if he totally believed in Jesus but there was something about the way he was spiritually that made me feel okay with that. Even if he didn't believe in Jesus the way I do, he was not trying to project his religion or his spirituality on to me. He said something like if God is not in the room, then he didn't want to be there either. That was cool with me. From a Christian point of view, I get that idea that we may come from different denominations, and my God could be different to the God you praise. But I liked that Wiremu wasn't trying to change anything within the situation spiritually that I might have been uncomfortable with.

One of the things that helped me about that session was that I felt more confident after meeting Wiremu that what we were doing was right for Grace. I'm not saying that we had all the answers. Meeting him affirmed for me that every path we took and every angle that we were looking at mattered. To me, you can't just work on one aspect of the person and not the rest. We were addressing the cultural point of view and the Christian point of view. We were considering the physical, the mental and the spiritual aspects. It wasn't to say that one was more important than the other. They all had to fit together.

The way we addressed Grace's spiritual wellbeing was through our prayers and through our church family. We attended to her mental wellbeing by coming to Health Pasifika and meeting Allister. I also focused on emotionally instilling it into her that it wasn't her fault. There was nothing that she had done to cause this. We paid attention to her physical wellbeing by ensuring that she was safe and that she felt safe. When she didn't feel safe at home, we moved to my Mum and Dad's place, where she did feel safe.

It felt like the session with Wiremu brought everything together for our family. We had Wiremu, our pastor, Allister and my Mum all in the room together. My only regret was that I didn't invite Grace's Dad. But he was able to attend an appointment with Allister a month later and hear about it. If he had been there and met Wiremu, he may have got a better understanding of what was going on for Grace. When he first found out, because he is Samoan, he suggested we take her to a Samoan healer. I don't think I would have felt comfortable with that. However, when I explained to him what Wiremu told us, I think he understood more. After hearing about this, he told me for the first time about times when he has felt spooked by some of his own spiritual experiences.

A key moment of the session with Wiremu was my realisation that the relationship problems between Grace's father and me were a huge part of why Grace was going through those experiences. I first thought about that after reading the story Allister gave me before the session (NiaNia et al., 2013). In that story I identified with the mum and the dad in that family, and I thought, wow! I could see how their breakup and behaviour towards each other had a role in their daughter's spiritual problem. Before that I was in denial about this matter. I was telling myself I wasn't doing anything wrong, and I was a great mother. I'm not saying I'm not. At the same time, now I think, yep, I'm not going to sit there and take all the blame for it, but I need to take responsibility for my part in it. I began to reflect on some of the shitty things I did, like projecting my feelings about their father onto my kids.

When Wiremu talked about what happens between parents affecting the young people, that made sense to me. It made it more concrete. He hit the nail on the head right there. After that I had to put my big girl pants on and try to move on and get over my anger with my ex-partner. Not to say that we are best of friends now. After that it took quite a bit of determination for me to calm down and listen to what he was saying, but I worked on that for the benefit of our kids. I think more than anything, once I changed the way I thought and felt about him, things started changing for Grace. After that she looked more comfortable around her Dad. I know she has always loved her Dad, but she and her sister were always on Mum's team. After the separation they were caught between us. Now when I feel angry with their Dad,

I just have to hold my tongue and talk to a friend later when they are not around, if I need to get it off my chest.

Women shouldn't have to put up with violence. And children shouldn't have to put up with parents saying horrible things about the other parent in front of them. I am continuing to address what happened between my ex-partner and me. I make sure the kids are safe and make sure that regardless of what he did, they know it wasn't their fault, and he's not angry with them. Their Dad has his own problems, and he needs to address them himself. We have been attending a Families Living Without Violence programme, and that's been helpful.

I liked what Wiremu said about spiritual authority. It starts with the head of the family. If I'm the head of our family, then I want to be a role model for what that authority looks like for our family. Wiremu said that if the spiritual authority of the family and the young person are both strong, then it's hard for these negative spiritual things to stick. If we can instil that authority in our children and grandchildren, then I hope they will be protected, and their wellbeing maintained.

Five Years after the Family Healing Session

Recently Allister contacted me and sent me a copy of this chapter. As I read through it for the first time, I couldn't help but shed some tears as I remembered this time. I was recalling how difficult it was for all of us. At the same time, I felt empowered by the story. I liked the way it shines a light on spirituality, the importance of spiritual authority and addressing unresolved hurts in the family. When I showed Grace the chapter, she was curious to read it. Her first response was to become tearful, just as I did. She asked me, 'How did that happen?' I told her it's nothing to be ashamed of, and she said, 'I'm not ashamed, Mum.' After we had talked about it for some time, she was able to acknowledge, 'You know Mum, that's my story!'

Grace will be 16 soon. Since that time just before meeting Wiremu, she has never had any more experiences of voices or visions. She works hard at school and enjoys hanging out with her friends. She is keen on her youth group and social media but is also comfortable with her own company. Overall, I would say in the last five years she hasn't looked back.

I also showed the story to Grace's Dad. Afterwards, I could see the sadness in his face. He didn't question any of it. I knew he was blaming himself for what we all went through. After getting out of jail, he saw several counsellors. At first, he just told them what he thought they wanted to hear. Later, he found a counsellor who didn't pussyfoot around and was very direct with him. With this counsellor, over a long period of time, he was able to look at some painful things from his own life. After that he had a stronger foundation for being a Dad with them. He felt more comfortable with himself, and as a result, his relationships with the girls improved. He gave up drinking a while ago and stopped hanging out with the guys he would socialise with before. He has had a steady job and has been working hard to improve who he is.

Six months ago, we got back together. It took me a very long time to trust him again. Once he took responsibility for what he did, over time I was able to acknowledge my part in what happened between us. When we first got together, I was 15 and he was 18. I was pregnant with Grace when I was very young. We are not teenagers anymore: we're adults. Neither of us are perfect. Every day we are working on our relationship and trying to be better than yesterday.

Wiremu

We have looked at Grace's problem of the voice and visions she experienced from multiple people's viewpoints. Her family tackled this problem from their Christian point of view, but they also asked for medical advice. Allister examined it from his child psychiatrist viewpoint and considered if it could be psychosis, trauma or another physical health cause. For me, I always look to wairua first. As well as the information I picked up from wairua, I was able to share concepts from te ao Māori to which the whānau responded with their own kōrero.

These diverse perspectives are not separate. It is harmful to say it's just one or the other. I am one person with all of these parts. The psychological hurt Grace experienced after witnessing her Dad assault her Mum could be considered a hinengaro (psychological) problem from one viewpoint, but it is intimately linked to her whānau and her tinana (body) and has profound negative effects on her wairua, as we have seen. If we as clinicians and wairua practitioners work together, we can offer a response that creates space for each of these. There is a saying, 'E hia kē ngā tāera waru kūmara.' There are many ways to peel a kūmara.

8 Jake

Wiremu NiaNia, Jake, Allister Bush, and David Epston

He kākano ahau i ruia mai i Rangiātea (I am a seed sown from Rangiātea)
(Whakatauākī – proverb)

Jake was 18 when he first met Wiremu. A talented singer and dancer, Jake was referred to the Māori Child, Adolescent and Family service (Māori CAFS) at Te Whare Mārie by the mental health crisis team after seriously harming himself. His Māori CAFS social worker asked if Jake could meet with Wiremu and Allister because he was puzzled by Jake's experiences of hearing voices without experiencing any other psychotic symptoms.[1]

This account begins by describing the background to Jake's referral to Māori CAFS and his two sessions with Allister and Wiremu, before giving Wiremu's perspectives on meeting Jake and his cultural explanation of Jake's experiences. It continues with reflections from Jake, Allister and Wiremu over the following 10 years.

Allister

Jake's First Session

Meeting Jake for the first time, my immediate impression was that he was wearing an unusual ensemble: a fashionable black leather jacket and pyjama trousers. What interested me was not so much that he was wearing pyjamas but that he had bothered to attend our meeting at all, given that he had so recently awoken. Responding to my curiosity, Jake said he'd stayed up late the previous night to farewell a friend who was leaving for overseas. After his mother, Heather, tried to rouse him for the third time 15 minutes before our 1 PM appointment time, he had been in a rush to leave the house.

Jake insisted that he wanted to meet with us privately, without his mother, and said their relationship had been strained in the lead-up to the

DOI: 10.4324/9781003187042-8

appointment. Willie, Jake's Māori CAFS social worker, introduced Jake to Wiremu and me and led us all through to the clinic room. Jake apologised for his attire but didn't seem self-conscious about it and said somewhat ruefully that he was still feeling the effects of a hangover from farewelling his friend.

Jake had met Willie twice over the previous week, and I had the impression they had hit it off pretty well. I also gathered that any motivation Jake had to attend our session was centred on his curiosity about Wiremu and an eagerness to find out what he might have to say or do.

Willie began the meeting by summarising some of the matters they had discussed at their previous sessions. He said Jake had considerable talent as a dancer and singer and was attending a local performing arts college. Jake's recent crisis had blown up on a day when he had been contemplating withdrawing from the programme to take up a new career opportunity. When Jake texted his father to tell him about this proposal, his father was clearly unimpressed. Over the next few hours, the exchange of texts between Jake and his father became increasingly heated. By the end of the day, Jake had become incensed with his father's attitude, and after several drinks, he began to feel even more enraged and despairing. At the height of this turmoil, Jake threw his cell phone across the room, breaking it. Infuriated with himself, Jake seized a knife from the kitchen in his flat and cut himself across his forearm. Jake's flatmate immediately intervened to take the knife away from him. When Jake's mother learned about this incident the next day, she had insisted Jake be referred for an assessment at our Māori CAFS service.

By the time Willie first met with him a day or so later, Jake regretted cutting himself and insisted he had no intention of ending his life. He said he had plenty of hopes for the future and, as far as he was concerned, 'The good always outweighs the bad.' He said alcohol had adversely affected his judgement and exaggerated his exasperation over his father's negative response to his plan to withdraw from his course.

Willie was satisfied that Jake didn't have significant symptoms of major depression. However, during Willie's routine enquiry about possible psychotic symptoms, Jake casually commented that he frequently heard voices. Sometimes they would offer him advice about what he was about to do. For example, he recalled the voices saying, 'Think about it' and 'Don't be an idiot', which he viewed as cautioning him against taking an unwise course of action. Sometimes he would hear a number of voices all together and couldn't always untangle one from the other. The voices would sometimes speak in te reo Māori (the Māori language), and when that happened, Jake didn't always understand them. The voices sometimes seemed to come from outside his head, but Jake wasn't clear on where they might be coming from. Interestingly, he had been having similar experiences for so long that he couldn't even remember when they began, although he suspected it was probably in his early primary school years. He was often curious about the voices but untroubled by them. He assumed they were some kind of spiritual experience.

As Jake had been having these experiences for a long time, they weren't associated with other psychotic symptoms, and he didn't appear troubled by them, Willie was fairly confident they didn't indicate the presence of a psychotic illness. However, he was keen for us to review them in light of Jake's recent episode of cutting himself.

During this first part of the interview, Wiremu interacted briefly with Jake but then remained mostly silent. He'd told me before the session that he wanted to get a feel for the situation and asked me to interview Jake as I usually would. After 40 minutes, Wiremu and Willie excused themselves as they had a prior commitment to attend. Wiremu asked Jake if he could visit him at Jake's home the following week, and Jake readily agreed. After they left, I continued to ask Jake about his life and experiences.

After a few minutes Jake sat back into his chair and assumed a more relaxed posture. When I asked him if he'd heard any voices recently, he said he'd heard quite a few voices before Wiremu left. He hadn't really understood what they were saying, but all the noise had ceased when Wiremu left the room. He said he felt calmer now as there seemed to have been a lot happening in the room when Wiremu was present. He also spoke about feeling sensations of itchiness that suggested to him that 'spiritual stuff' was going on.

I was curious about Jake's experience of Wiremu and struck by how self-assured he seemed to be in his view that the voices he'd heard in the past were likely to be spiritual in nature. I began to ask him in detail about other spiritual experiences he could recall.

Jake began to talk about a wide range of similar experiences over almost the entire course of his life. The first incident he mentioned happened before he was old enough to remember it: he had heard about it second-hand. When it happened, Jake's parents were no longer living together. Jake had become severely ill after two days of flu-like symptoms, and when his mother sought a medical assessment at an after-hours medical centre, he was rushed to hospital by ambulance. After Jake was admitted to the paediatric ward, his condition continued to deteriorate. To Heather's horror, he became so pale and floppy that he was considered to be near death. Heather maintained her overnight vigil beside Jake's bed, but briefly fell asleep in the early hours of the morning. Shortly afterwards she was woken by what felt like a person beside her, even though there didn't appear to be anyone else physically present in the room. Heather wasn't afraid but was aware she was not alone.

When Heather told Jake's paternal aunt about this experience the next day, his aunt said it was very likely to have been a protective visit from Jake's paternal grandmother, whom Jake referred to as his Nanny. His Nanny had died many years before. Jake's aunty believed his Nanny visited Jake and Heather to support them. She had also felt his Nanny's presence that night but didn't know why until Heather phoned her the next day to share her experience. After a lumbar puncture, Jake was diagnosed with meningitis and treated with antibiotics, and went on to make a full recovery.

Heather was Pākehā (New Zealand European), and Jake's father was Māori. When Jake was four years old, Heather and Jake's paternal grandfather, whom Jake called 'Koro', took him to visit his father's tūrangawaewae or family land in the far north to learn about his whakapapa (genealogy). When they visited the urupā (burial ground) on the hill behind the marae (meeting house), Jake had become very excited and began running amongst the gravestones. When Heather finally caught up with Jake he was standing by the grave of his paternal great-grandfather and 'throat singing' a sad keening song in ancient te reo Māori, using words he couldn't possibly have known and that were very different to the songs he learned in kōhanga reo (Māori language preschool). Heather tried to pick him up and console him, but he resisted her and clung to the graveside, digging his fingers into the soil, until he had finished. Afterwards, Jake clambered up into his mother's arms and seemed more peaceful.

Jake recalled that he had always been tall for his age and stood out because he was taller than most of his whānau (family). His paternal great-grandfather had also been tall, similar in appearance to Jake, with a darker complexion and a quiet and often serious demeanour.

During his primary school years, Jake had been known for his sparky ideas. If one of these ideas gripped his imagination, he would pursue it vigorously at the earliest possible moment without regard for potential danger or pitfalls. In fact, his tendency to follow his impulses and some difficulties he had paying attention in class in his early years had led one paediatrician to suggest he had a form of attention deficit hyperactivity disorder (ADHD). However, Jake had no time for this notion, and although he was prescribed treatment for ADHD, he decided not to continue with it. Nevertheless, it did seem that the cautionary advice Jake had been given by his voices had spared him from many sticky situations over the years.

Jake confided in a member of his father's whānau, who told him the voices could be ancestors. In particular, it was suggested that Jake's Nanny and great-grandfather were keeping a close eye on his progress and were very likely to be the voices of caution he would hear from time to time. This idea was a source of comfort to Jake and enhanced his sense of belonging to his father's whānau, despite long absences between seeing his father.

At times he would experience these voices as loving and supportive, which he said confirmed the kinship connection he felt with them.

Jake also talked about knowing things that he couldn't know through normal means of communication. For example, he would suddenly feel grief-stricken and have a foreboding that someone close to him had died. His intuition would frequently be confirmed later on. Sometimes he could recall seeing or feeling something like a spiritual presence in the room. When I asked him more about these kinds of experiences, he found them very difficult to put words to. However, such experiences felt very familiar to him and not unpleasant.

As Jake spoke, I was thinking about possible psychiatric explanations for his unusual experiences. His voices could have been auditory hallucinations, perhaps a symptom of a psychotic illness. But rather than being bothered by the voices, Jake described them as loving and supportive at times. The fact that Jake's voices dated back to early childhood and that they weren't accompanied by other psychotic symptoms such as disorganised thinking or delusions also counted against a psychotic illness hypothesis. The voices certainly didn't seem to have had a disabling effect on Jake's life. Given Jake's view of the voices as spiritual experiences, I was curious to hear Wiremu's perspective on this question.

Towards the end of the session, Jake and I reviewed a number of situations in which drinking alcohol had led to circumstances that Jake later regretted. Jake seemed to reflect on these moments openly but didn't want to change his drinking habits. Having confirmed Willie's view that Jake had no further intent to harm himself, I agreed with Jake that we would meet Wiremu at Jake's flat the following week.

The Second Session, at Jake's Flat

When Wiremu and I arrived at Jake's flat a week later, Jake was waiting to meet us in the driveway. We entered his house through a sliding door directly into the living area. He invited Wiremu and me to sit on the couch opposite the door, while he took the easy chair just inside the door. To our left was a door that led to bedrooms in the flat. The winter sun was shining into the room from behind Jake, and his guitar was propped up next to him.

After Jake welcomed us, Wiremu asked Jake whom he was living with and, shortly afterwards, made a reference to some spiritual entities in the room with us. I was nonplussed to hear Jake confirm Wiremu's observation and point out where in the room he could sense three entities. He pointed to a corner of the room to the left of where Wiremu and I were sitting. Wiremu confirmed the location of this entity and said he was concerned it might be related to the mother of Jake's flatmate, who was also living in the house. He urged Jake to take care of himself around this person. Wiremu then said he could sense two kaitiaki (guardians) next to Jake, and Jake corroborated that he was aware of their presence and had a fair idea which of his deceased ancestors they were.

At this point Wiremu invited Jake to sing one of his own songs for us. Jake agreed without hesitation, picked up his guitar and gave us a rousing rendition of his latest composition. I was struck by his obvious technical skill on the acoustic guitar and his passionate vocal performance. In a moment, he was totally immersed in the music. His next song conjured up a more soulful atmosphere. When Jake put his guitar down, Wiremu and I marvelled at his accomplished performance and Wiremu asked if he planned to record his compositions. Wiremu then commented that Jake had been in a relationship with an older woman and again urged caution, encouraging Jake to take care of himself when it came to affairs of the heart. He warned him that cannabis and other substances would be very dangerous for him due to his spiritual awareness and openness. Jake accepted Wiremu's offer to finish our session with a karakia (prayer).

Wiremu

The first time I met Jake, at our workplace, there were different things going on around him. The tīpuna (ancestors) who were with us were interacting, and so of course it could have sounded noisy to him.

When we met with Jake at his flat, it was different. This time there was a flurry of activity but not a lot of noise. I could feel three distinct entities in the room. And Jake could feel them as well. When I mentioned them, he pointed to where they were in the room. The one that I saw out to my left was a female presence, so I asked Jake who else was staying in the house. He said that his flatmate's mother had come to stay. As he said that, I noticed a headache that gripped my head and felt she had issues that could affect him negatively. Therefore, I said to him, 'Don't get involved in any stuff she might pour out.' Sometimes people can have emotional stuff that they hold in their puku (stomach) and it's as if they spew it out onto the carpet. I was thinking it could splash on Jake, and he could be infected by those spiritual germs.

There were two other entities there. There was an older woman, a kuia, close to the left of him. When I mentioned her, Jake acknowledged her as his Nanny. There was a male presence on his right who was very laid-back and quiet. I felt reassured that Jake was safe, with the kuia on his left and the koroua on his right. He was comfortable with their presence. So that is the appropriate side for female and male to be. They were quiet and dignified, but this other female presence to my left-hand side was flitting around in an unsettling way. However, I noticed that it seemed to be keeping its distance from the kuia who was on Jake's left side and the koroua on his right. The kuia would move a little and then return to his side while the other entity seemed to be trying to find a gap in their defence but was clearly unable to do so. In terms of protecting Jake, it wasn't aggressive, just a natural protection, like covering Jake in a korowai (protective cloak).

Given this protection, I felt somewhat reassured about Jake's wellbeing. I didn't think he was going to need a lot of help relating to wairua (spiritual realm). However, there was a 'but'. If he got into a close relationship and then there was a split, I had this feeling a break-up could be a very painful thing for him that might hurt his heart. I worried that drugs and alcohol under those circumstances could be very dangerous for him. That's the sort of feeling I was getting from the kuia and the koroua. I was sure that was why they were keeping a close eye on him.

When I consider the detail of Jake's experiences, he talked of hearing voices coming from outside of himself and counselling him with sound advice. They could be critical but not nasty: more like parent figures. He talked about them speaking in te reo Māori, using expressions he didn't always understand. To me, this is consistent with voices from tīpuna. Meeting him at his flat and having my own experience of the kuia and koroua next to him confirmed this. He could feel them there. This shared experience with Jake allowed me to verify his experience with my own. If he doubted himself, I was able to reassure him. It also allowed me to advise any clinician who might be working with him that this was a wairua experience rather than psychosis or another psychiatric symptom. I gave an example of such a shared experience in Chapter 1, when I told the story of what happened at Parikanapa station.

There is another aspect of Jake's experience that I wish to comment on. After our second meeting, Allister asked me about Jake's difficulties putting words to his experiences of wairua. Allister might ask him, 'Was it like a voice that you were hearing?' and Jake would say, 'No, that's not quite it.' And it seemed that for Jake, it was more that he sensed something was there rather than seeing it. He described it as if he was feeling something there with a part of his brain.

This difficulty expressing wairua in words is very familiar to me. In sensing wairua, it often seems to me that I hear things with my vision or see things with my hearing or taste things with my eyes. In our language there is a saying: 'Kei te rongo au te kakara o te kai.' Literally, this means 'I can hear the fragrance of the food.' Or someone might say, 'Kei te rongo au te reka o te kai,' which means, 'I can hear the sweet taste of the food.' From my perspective, all the senses are connected. Everything is interconnected.

The message for Jake in this situation was from his kuia and koroua. Even though he was already aware of their presence, they were reminding him of their tautoko (support) and korowai. In my view, the other female presence had no message for him; she just happened to be there. The whakapapa connection for Jake is obvious: the kuia and koroua are his tīpuna. The significance for Jake of becoming aware of this connection shouldn't be underestimated. In Chapter 6 with Tohu, we saw the impact that such a connection can have. With regard to the female entity on my left in his flat, the only connection to Jake was that her wairua was in the living area of his whare (house). She had a connection to his flatmate, but not to him. The fruit of this experience for Jake is that he gets to know the richness of his whakapapa line. It is a living demonstration of his identity as part of that genealogical tree. He is a seed of this line. The whakatauākī which we referred to at the outset of this chapter begins, 'He kākano ahau, i ruia mai e Rangiātea.' 'He kākano' refers to a seed, and 'Rangiātea' is the original heavenly space alluding to our belief that ultimately we are descended from divinity. This whakatauākī reminds us that we all come from long lines of female and male rangatira or chiefs. Even in our most despairing moments, this proverb reminds us that we are part of something bigger: that we have an intimate connection to all those who came before us.

All parts of that whakapapa tree are important. Every seed matters. Tohunga whakairo or master carvers have a karakia they recite when they are about to cut down a majestic tree in the forest. After felling the tree, they take care to gather all the branches and all the foliage. Then when they have completed their carving, they collect all the wood chips and sawdust they carved out of the trunk of that tree. Every part is gathered up and buried with appropriate ritual and karakia. Nothing is overlooked. In the same way, everyone has an important place in their whakapapa and will not be forgotten.

So, if we consider all these matters and return to a key theme of this book, we can ask the question: What is the nature of the voices that Jake was sensing? In these situations, I'm observing matters very closely. It's a fine line to discern what is spiritual and what is not. It's hard for me to reach any sort of conclusion unless I can hear the voice myself or discern the source of that voice, so I won't make a call if I have any doubts at all. If I do make a call, I'm confident about what it is that I'm picking up. And during our meeting with Jake, it became clear to me that he was having spiritual experiences and that he was perceiving the same entities in the room at the same time that I was. This convinced me that the voices he could hear were likely to be spiritual in origin rather than psychiatric or psychological.

Returning to the session with Jake at his flat; near the end, something interesting happened. Jake made a comment about his mother warning him about getting into sexual relationships too early, and he said something very dismissive about his mum's concern. Just as he said that I suddenly saw very clearly a woman. This woman, although a young adult, was definitely older than him. So, I said, 'Not the older woman, I hope!' and he laughed and said 'Yeah, she was 21.' I'm not sure why I was shown this, but perhaps it served to build a bit of rapport with him. When he acknowledged that she was 21, I knew that I'd got through to him. And it wasn't too long after that he said, 'Oh, I wouldn't mind seeing you again.'

Later in our session, Jake spoke about getting a feeling about something that was going on for someone and using that information to play a trick on them. That is an experience that I know about. Because he has that capacity to know stuff that he shouldn't know, he's tempted to use that knowledge to play with their heads. It's not in a malicious way. Those tricks can feel beautiful because others are mystified by what's going on. But sometimes people don't realise that games like that can have serious consequences. So, I'm very careful about the privacy of others these days and wouldn't use my knowledge mischievously or maliciously. I have come to learn this through trial and error. and I'm sure Jake will do the same in time.

Kaitiaki

Tiaki means to protect. Kai means that someone is in the process of doing something. So, someone who is a kaitiaki can be compared to a mentor. They are watching over someone and are a guardian for that person. For example, angels are kaitiaki: they're guardians. In Aotearoa, iwi (tribes) are usually kaitiaki for the moana (sea), awa (rivers) and whenua (land) in their local area. Spiritual kaitiaki offer the same kind of protection. Often, they come from the same whakapapa line, but not always. I've known people who had kaitiaki who were not their ancestors. Perhaps it was someone who had a special interest or concern for them who may have assumed the role of a kaitiaki. If they were someone who cared for injured animals, then they could attract a kaitiaki who had acted similarly during their lifetime on earth and then became available to them as their kaitiaki. Frequently, however, kaitiaki are from the same whānau. In fact, families often have certain kaitiaki who help and may warn particular family members in times of danger. I believe this to be the case for Jake. I have several kaitiaki myself.

Kaitiaki may warn you in times of danger, but sometimes people who don't know about them and their purposes may find them confusing or distressing. It's not unusual for young people to experience this if they don't have sufficient understanding. Some people are fortunate enough to have pakeke or elders who can guide them and explain that their tīpuna are here to assist them in difficult times. In te ao Māori (the Māori world), kaitiaki are commonly accepted (Benton et al., 2013; Moon, 2003; NiaNia et al., 2017, 2019). Certainly, this knowledge has been around my whānau for generations, and we still live by that.

Two Years after the First Session

Jake

I remember the day I met with Wiremu and Allister in my flat, even though it was a while ago. I was sitting on the blue couch, and I recall Wiremu talking about other people being there with us. I could feel them there as well. There was one on my right side, one on my left side, and another one away from me off to my right.

The two people close to me are often there. I've been told by my aunty that they are ancestors. One is my great-grandfather on my Dad's side, who apparently looked rather like me. She also said that his wife, my great-grandmother, is sometimes around me. However, I'm not really aware of her presence. I believe that the older woman who Wiremu saw next to me in my flat was my Nanny, my Dad's mother. I often feel her there. I believe that she decided to watch over me more closely after I got meningitis when I was young. That makes sense to me because my Dad was one of 13 kids and he got meningitis when he was very small. His brother also contracted meningitis and was severely disabled after that. It was around that time that my grandmother died suddenly. And because she wasn't able to protect her children from the meningitis, I believe that's why she came to me when meningitis was about to destroy us again. Often in my life I've heard their voices talking to me. Many times they have said something reassuring and they back each other up. Other times they'll tell me what's right and what's wrong. For example, they might say, 'Don't have that extra drink.' I know that it's for my own good even if I feel irritated at the time.

Hearing Wiremu describing these same people being there and knowing I could feel them there too, I remember feeling quite content with myself. To hear this coming from someone who is quite spiritual really backed up what I was experiencing. It made me feel less crazy. Trying to accept spirituality isn't easy. People try to find a medical reason. I don't think I'm crazy, but sometimes I doubt myself. Sitting there with Wiremu, I just remember feeling really calm. Perhaps what helped me was that he was giving me time to understand, or maybe it was that he really did understand what I was talking about.

Later in our meeting, Wiremu mentioned that I had a relationship with an older woman. He was right about that. When I read his comments in this chapter about me being vulnerable to a relationship break-up, he was exactly right about that, too. Not long after I saw him, a girl whom I had been very close with for a long time, whom I considered to be my soulmate and who was overseas, told me she was with someone else. It pretty much destroyed my life. I stayed in my room for two weeks solid, drinking and smoking. Finally, my flatmate brought round most of my friends and insisted that I come out of my room. It's exactly what Wiremu had predicted. This is why hearing this buzzed me out so much because what he said about me was really true. I've had two serious relationships since then, and I got very emotional in both situations when they broke up.

I was interested in what Wiremu said about how perceiving spiritual things is not exactly feeling, and not seeing or hearing, but perhaps a mixture of those experiences. I can quite often feel people's emotions. In fact, that's probably one of the strongest spiritual experiences I have. When I'm talking to friends, and being there in the conversation, sometimes I can 'hear' their distress, even though they're not expressing it openly. I can literally hear crying, when they might not be letting on that they are sad or upset or when they are trying to cover it up. But I can hear that feeling that they are having. Or at other times I can feel that strong emotion in the room, like anger. Other times I can hear what they are saying behind the words. I may experience this in sound as little grunts, or little angry sounds. These are some of the different ways I know the feelings that others aren't expressing directly to me.

Every human being is spiritual. Some of us have developed it more, just as Wiremu said. Pacific people have and of course we as Māori have. But I know that Pākehā also have this spiritual awareness. However, for many it is hard to accept the spiritual. With the physical world, the real things are more obvious. Like this phone is real, or that drink can is real. But some people might say that the extra people in this room around us aren't real. I know that's not true because they are just as real as you and me. And being with someone like Wiremu really helps me because he is able to confirm these experiences. They are there. You can't grab them. You can't talk to them the way you and I are talking. But they are real all right.

Allister

As Jake had not been suffering from a significant mental health problem at the time we first met and didn't need further assistance from a mental health service, he was soon discharged. When I contacted Jake two years later, I told him about our proposal to write about those first meetings with Wiremu. Jake was enthusiastic about this idea and wanted to meet up. I could tell that he was particularly keen to see Wiremu again.

We arranged to pick him up in the central city, and he took us to a local youth centre, where we caught up on his news. Just as before, I was struck by his exuberance and energy. He was bursting with ideas, experiences and music. At our invitation he grabbed a guitar lying against a wall. His performance of his own songs was as passionate and skilfully crafted as it had been two years before. Although we were not meeting in a clinical setting, Jake was very open about how things had been going for him. When

I enquired about his recent experiences, I was satisfied that, from a psychiatric point of view, while Jake continued to have the same experiences of voices, visions and feelings from time to time, he had no other symptoms indicating a mental health problem. However, I was concerned about what he said about his recent heavy alcohol and drug use and the effects this could have on his wellbeing.

Wiremu

I enjoyed meeting Jake again, but I was concerned because I could feel that he had been using drugs that could be very harmful for him. And as we were sitting in the room with him, I was aware of a few entities there. There was a woman who clearly showed herself to me. She was sitting in a chair just to Jake's right. It was obvious to me that she was very distinguished. She was dressed in elegant clothes, including a black blouse with white trim. Her hair was long and carefully tied back like a ponytail, but perhaps more sophisticated than a ponytail. She felt to me like a very lovely woman. She was just quietly observing Jake and what was going on. She wasn't making any facial expressions or anything like that but rather was just sitting there. She had olive skin, but it wasn't apparent to me if she was Māori or Pākehā. Usually I have an inkling as to why they are there, but this time I couldn't tell why. She appeared to be just sitting as if to say, 'I am here.' I was sure that she was like a kaitiaki for Jake, and she'd probably been there with him over a period of years. It was interesting to me that she was sitting on his right as usually the women are on the left of a person. Sometimes that can mean that they are connected to the male line. However, that's how it was.

Jake has great talent as a singer and songwriter, and I appealed to him to take care of this as a way to engage him in thinking about his drug use. Drinking so much alcohol and using drugs in the way he was doing can be harmful, particularly for those with spiritual gifts. In Chapter 5, I talked about how mind-altering substances can wedge open spiritual doorways for people and alter their ability to maintain control over their own experiences.

Jake's gift tells me that he has the potential to help others in the future. At the same time his spiritual and musical gifts can lead to unexpected pitfalls. They could result in him being led into trouble by his pride, his ego. We all have this ego, and it can easily trip us up. My ego can make me believe that this gift I have is really me, and that I am such a great person. In feeling puffed up like this, I can end up saying things to others that put them down or dismiss them, and there lies the danger. Such actions can come back on me in a worldly way or in a spiritual way. If I'm not careful to tame my ego, to keep control over it, I can lose what I have in terms of a gift, whether that be a spiritual or even a musical gift. I could get ill, perhaps dangerously ill, or someone in my family could get ill. In Jake's case, if his ego runs away with him, then he could easily hurt someone else's feelings without intending to, or put others down, or cause them to feel jealous of him. And if this happened then the unseen in others could take offense, and he could be in for a rough ride. It's all right to feel confident but very important not to be cocky. It's essential to remain humble in order to take care of ourselves spiritually.

Three-and-a-Half Years after the First Session

Jake

I have enjoyed reading Wiremu and Allister's reflections from our last contact about 18 months ago. The woman he described seeing beside me resembles exactly a photo that I have seen of my Nanny some time before she died. Also, Wiremu's predictions about the problems I could fall into with alcohol and drugs, and then later his concerns about my drug use, were spot on. When we last met, that was a time when I was indulging in a lot of drugs that I probably shouldn't have done. It's now a year since I cut down my drug use quite drastically. When I turned 21, one of the big wake-up calls for me was having my little kaitiaki talk to me: my brother and sister, who are flesh-and-blood kaitiaki. My brother told me, 'I love hanging out with you, except when you are on drugs.' He was 17 at the time. I would like to think of myself as a good influence for my brother and sister, but they were telling me that the good influence came from the sober Jake, not the wasted Jake. I've grown up my whole life trying to decipher what's real and what's not real. For me being real is a big thing. I began to realise that my brother, seeing me drunk, was beginning to think that my claims that I cared for him were fake and not real. That inspired a massive change in my outlook.

I'm still experiencing a lot of spiritual things every day, but the advice that I used to enjoy getting is much less now. It's as if they feel they can let me go now to make my own decisions. The kaitiaki are giving me more space. That's a bit scary and a bit sad for me sometimes. There were times in the past when I used to love to be alone so that I could talk with them. For example, when I was, say, 13 or 14, I would be alone and I would put a thought out there, and I might get seven or eight responses. I loved having a 60-year-old point of view coming at me. Some of the responses were strong, some not. Some were heartfelt, some not. That's how I would decipher who they were. The sad thing is that now they are still there but all I hear is 'you know' and 'carry on,' which is encouraging I guess, but I used to really appreciate the detailed advice. The fact is I do know that they will always be there but perhaps they are letting me know that I have the strength to stand on my own now. Maybe I don't need the korowai in the same way.

Often now, when I have these spiritual experiences, it almost seems as if it's not for me. It seems to be for others. That's what I thought was cool about what Wiremu said about helping others. I can also relate to what Wiremu said about being careful about ego. In the past the voices would say things like, 'Calm down, that's your ego, shut up!' Now they don't. Perhaps they have a sense that I'm starting to have more awareness of that. I still frequently notice positive and negative spiritual things around people or in different places. I will avoid some places because of that. But there is something else that has changed for me. I have become more accepting of those negative spiritual things. Instead of just ignoring them, sometimes I will try to be accepting of them. For example, I might notice one and say to myself, 'Oh well, you are coming here, but this isn't anywhere you can stop, so just keep going!' I think that every spirit, even the cold ones, even the bad ones, need to be healed. They all have something to learn.

Ten Years after the First Session

Allister

While writing this chapter I contacted Jake for an update on his life and experiences. At this time the world was in the midst of the COVID-19 pandemic, and New Zealand was in lockdown, with almost everyone confined to their homes. I spoke to Jake over the internet by video. He explained that he was training in youth work and thoroughly enjoying it. Listening to him and looking at him, I could tell he was thriving. In the intervening years, Jake had several times briefly sought support from mental health services. Each time he was distressed in relation to life circumstances, including a relationship break-up and the birth of a child. At no time had he seen a mental health clinician about any concerns related to psychosis.

Jake read through this chapter at my request and had one correction to make. He explained that during the incident with the knife, he had stabbed himself in the wrist, rather than cutting himself. He described it as an immediate reaction and pulled up his sleeve to show me the scar. Other than that, he told me, 'The rest of the story is spot on.'

In the following section Jake talks about his experience of tīpuna and other voices and visions ten years after first meeting Wiremu, and how he now makes sense of these experiences.

Jake

Looking back, my understanding about wairua has changed in many ways. I still have wairua experiences every day. Frequently I see or hear things I can't explain. In the past I would want an immediate answer to what was happening. Now I am more comfortable with uncertainty. Sometimes the answer may be another question, or another thought; it is hardly ever a solid answer. I more often accept what comes, even with the raw emotion that may accompany it.

With regards to my tīpuna, I am aware of three who are often with me. These days it is my Koro and Nanny whose presence I am aware of most often. The other one who is with me all the time is my great-grandfather.

My Koro passed away when I was 11, and in recent years it seems like he is constantly there with me. I generally feel him just behind my right shoulder. One way I recognise him is by how he feels. His energy – that feeling of aroha (love), patience and tautoko – is very familiar to me from being with him when I was young. I remember his voice in life as being deep and calm in tone. Now I hear it mostly in my mind, in which case it doesn't sound exactly the same. Occasionally, when I hear his voice out loud, it sounds a lot like his voice when I was little, but I still hear it as if it's coming from inside my head. His words and phrases have always been very distinctive. He preferred to use a poetic and slightly formal style in his kōrero (talk). For example, he might have said, 'Much water has flowed under the bridge since last we talked' and I would think, 'Well, that's a long-winded way of saying hello!' He still talks just like that. We share this love for beautiful words: me in lyrics I choose in my songwriting and him in the way he speaks to me.

His sense of humour is just as it always was. He laughs at things I find funny, but also at things I find hard to accept in myself. I may feel irritated by that, but I know he does it with love, just as he did when he was alive. Back then, even though I only saw him from time to time, every time I felt very connected to him, as if he was always there.

One of my aunties is very aware of wairua, and we have lots of conversations. She tells me that my Koro visits her regularly and she sees him often with me. She tells me that since he passed away, 'It's like he disappeared from this world and went and perched on your shoulder.'

I have lots of internal chats with my Koro and Nanny about ego. It's been huge for me. I think it was a big thing for my Koro as well. Certainly ten years ago I was caught up with my ego. It was clouding my vision. I wanted to be famous and change the world. Now I try to stop being so proud and act with a bit more humility. It's not easy for me. I have had to notice my ego, respect it and then let go of it. I realise it is a major part of me and my whakapapa. While that cockiness has been a problem for me, it has been the downfall of others in my whānau as well. When my Koro and I have these chats, I can hear him as both words and thoughts. His process of thought is not like my style of thought. As I described before with what he says, my grandfather's thoughts seem distinctly him, quite distinguishable to me from my own ways of thinking.

Allister asked me how I would distinguish the voice of my grandfather from a psychotic voice. I presume that a psychotic voice would be, by definition, harmful. My grandfather's voice is not harmful. If anything, it's the opposite: it gives me strength.

I once had an unmistakable experience of hearing a psychotic voice. It was in my early 20s, and I had used LSD. During one bad trip I felt like there was a terrible amount of evil in the world, and I was searching for answers. Suddenly a voice was yelling at me, 'Everything is shit!' It seemed like this voice was coming from inside my head. Even though I felt terrible, part of me knew that this was a product of my mind. Normally when I hear a voice talking to me when no living person is there, I can see or feel a spiritual entity to explain it. That time, there was no spiritual energy. That is one way I distinguish between psychotic and wairua experiences.

On the other hand, sometimes wairua and psychotic problems can go together. Last year a friend of mine developed a psychotic illness. He and I grew up together, and have stayed close. I knew he had been smoking weed in the six months before he became unwell. He is also open to spiritual energies, just as I am. When I was young, and I could see things in the wairua, sometimes he would see them too. I recognised he was psychotic from what he was saying. His talking was fast and mixed up. He would start with one sentence and then skip to another and perhaps end up back at the first sentence. His responses seemed irrelevant to what I was talking to him about or what was going on around him. He also was making some unrealistic calls about people's intentions and accused people of doing things they hadn't done. Sometimes he got very aggressive and lashed out at those around him.

Even though I accepted he was psychotic and supported his family in asking for help from mental health services, I also knew he had a spiritual problem too. I could feel this black, dense energy around him. It didn't feel good. It felt to me like that black spiritual entity was having a strong influence on him in a negative way. However, he wasn't able to get help with that wairua side. He had psychiatric treatment in hospital and a number of things improved, but I could still detect the negative entity there with him even six months after he went home from hospital.

These days, sometimes I am able to use my wairua experiences to help others make sense of their situation. For example, last week, I was talking to a friend on a video chat due to the lockdown. During our conversation she asked me what colour her aura was. Usually I don't talk to friends about wairua, because people often don't understand. However, some people question me about spirituality without any prompting. I don't always see auras or colours around people. But in this situation, even though we were in totally different places and communicating over the internet, for some reason I could see colours around her. I told her that the colour of her aura was yellow with some green. She said that people had previously told her that her aura was yellow, like a bright sun. But no one had commented on a green colour. She asked me, 'What's the green?' I had to think about it, I said, 'I don't know. It's not you.' At that moment, I realised that this green colour was somebody else's energy. We were both trying to figure out where it had come from. She then told me the story of the house that she was living in. It was sold due to the death of a teenager in the family. It transpired that she was sleeping in the room where he had also slept. His energy felt to me like 14 to 16 years old. When I explained my impression to her, the weird part about that was that I noticed she suddenly seemed to get defensive. As if she was responding, 'No, there is nobody there.' But alongside that, I heard him say, 'No, don't look at me.'

Allister

Curious to hear Jake describe his experience of this voice in more detail, I interrupted him to say, 'Please tell me more about your experience at that moment.' Jake paused to consider before replying. 'When I was interacting with him, I could feel his energy; I knew there was an entity there. Even though this is the first time I have felt something like this through a screen. But in saying that, once I could feel him there, it was almost as though he was here with me in this room. I physically heard him say, "I'm not here."'

I urged Jake, 'Could you describe more about that?' Jake paused again to reflect. He looked at me and I could tell he was concentrating hard. 'I'm not used to putting these things into words.' He took another breath and looked away, then turned back to face me. 'I realise this might sound strange, but I could hear his words in my body; in my stomach and my spine to be exact. I could feel him as if he was two or three metres in front of me, just to my right. He was there, but I heard his words inside my body. I couldn't ignore it.

> At that point I realised that this entity didn't want me to notice him. All at once, I could feel his sadness. I felt quite okay myself at that moment, but his presence brought the weight of sadness onto me. It came to me that he was just looking for somewhere he could be loved, thought about and cared for. I had the impression that he was justifying himself thinking, "I'm not hurting anybody." That's true, I thought. However, he didn't realise that he was having an emotional effect on her relationship with her own child and other aspects of her life. His control was subtly apparent in her decision-making. Even though he wasn't hurting her, she wasn't his. He didn't need to be there. His energy was not what I would call evil. Those ones are very apparent to me. He was just hurting. He was lonely, he said. He wasn't ready to go. That's understandable. Death

is a crazy thing. I don't think many are ever ready for it. At such a young age I can just imagine how you would want to remain. So I got talking to this boy and we got to this understanding that he was sad.

I interrupted Jake again. 'Please say more about what you mean about talking to him.' Jake gave me a puzzled look and thought for a moment.

I'm not used to explaining this. I was talking out loud to this guy because I wanted my friend to hear what I was saying to him. Eventually, I told him, "You're not a bad guy, but you're not allowed to be here, bro, sorry." After we reached that understanding, my friend started sobbing, but in a loving way. I think there was healing for her in this interaction. I was able to talk to the boy and say, "Actually we do need you to go, but go in love." After that she told me she felt like a weight had lifted. A few days later she told me, "Man, I have been feeling quite raw and open," which I took to mean spiritually open. I advised her to be careful. When you are open, it leaves space for things to come and latch on. She told me about a pīwakawaka (fantail) that had flown into her house that day. Often, a pīwakawaka flying into your house is interpreted in te ao Māori as a bad omen, but I realised in this case it was more of an assurance that she was very open at that moment.

Wiremu

In reading Jake's account of how he helped his friend, I noticed the way he described his role in their kōrero. He told that story in a matter-of-fact way. His focus seemed to be on helping her. Such a gift is there for a purpose, and I knew he had the potential to use this gift to help others once he found a way to tone down his ego. Others can easily be turned off by your self-importance. Spiritually, it's the same. There is no room for bragging in relation to Wairua.[2] However, if I say to Wairua, 'This person needs healing, and I come to you in all humility to ask for it,' then Wairua can flow. We are not the healers. We are just like hoses, through which the healing effects of Wairua can flow. The water or Wairua running though does not come from me. It comes from the Source. Ego can be like a blockage in that hose. It will get in the way of that flow of Wairua.

Alongside dealing with his ego, Jake had to address the role substances have played in his life. Many people with wairua gifts become sidetracked by addictions, and their gifts can be lost. Jake could have easily been ensnared in that way if he hadn't tackled that problem in his life.

Finally, I would like to comment on what Jake said about perceiving his friend's aura over the internet and his experience of the boy. This type of situation is very familiar to me. I'm not at all surprised that Jake could have that experience at a distance. This comes back to the meaning of wairua, which I outlined in Chapter 1. Wairua transcends all time and space. It's not dependent on being next to the person, although you do need some connection to them. It's the same way with being connected to Te Kaihanga, the Source. God is not limited by time and space. So it makes sense to me that healing for Jake's friend could have come about through that online connection at that moment.

Allister

In closing our video meeting, I asked Jake if he would like us to finish with karakia. He said he would like that. There was a pause as we both considered who might do the karakia. Then Jake spoke up. 'I've got one, if you want.' I was pleased to accept his offer. Jake went on, 'This is freestyle, by the way.'

There was a further pause as he collected his thoughts, then he said,

> Ki a koe te hau, ki a koe te ora, ngā hau e whā, piki mai, kake mai, i roto i tō mana te ora, whakamaua tōku kawa tōku mana i roto e tū. Ngā mihi mō te hā, mō te ao nui, mō te aroha, amene.

Translating for me, he said, 'This is a prayer to Tāwhirimātea (Atua of wind), about being the air, coming from the four corners of our world. This karakia talks about his journey of helping his brother Tāne[3] and helping humankind grow in our understanding of how the world works. I thanked him for being the breath, "te hā", the foundation of life. Without "hā" we can't live.'

Notes

1 Jake's story has been previously published as a case report in a psychiatric journal (NiaNia et al., 2019).
2 Wairua here refers to Divine Source.
3 Tāne here refers to Tānenuiārangi, a Māori atua who ascended the heavens to collect the three baskets of knowledge, with the assistance of his elder brother Tāwhirimātea. However, Jake also interprets Tāne in this context as referring to humankind.

9 Ngā Kūaha

Wiremu NiaNia and Allister Bush

Wiremu

For me, seeing, hearing or feeling something or someone in wairua (the spiritual realm) may be likened to the opening of a spiritual doorway or portal. This could be deliberate on my part or may occur unexpectedly. It may be welcome or it may be distressing. Such entranceways are what I refer to as ngā kūaha. When people seek my assistance about confusing or distressing voices, visions and other perceptions, I'm interested to understand whether their experiences relate to the opening up of such doorways.

In this chapter, I describe my approach to meeting people with such experiences. I'm not saying that these whakaaro (ideas) are the best or only approaches. Other people have their own ways. In the following chapter, Allister will offer his perspective on ways that mental health clinicians and others might recognise wairua experiences and identify when referral to a Māori healer or other wairua practitioner would be helpful.

Tātaihono is an approach to working together that involves deep mutual respect and inviting space for the views of the other to be considered and appreciated (NiaNia et al., 2017a). We have cultural and clinical approaches. We have wairua practitioners and clinicians. It's like having two hands. Whatever our task, it makes sense to use both hands together. It's not sensible to use one hand to do all the heavy lifting and leave the other hand out entirely. The left hand doesn't say 'I'm the boss' and exclude the right hand. They work together. I liken our two methods, my wairua approach to voices and visions and Allister's psychiatric approach, to these two hands. I believe that both roles are important and complementary. We need to find a balance between our different approaches.

Hui

I generally start a hui (meeting) with mihimihi, greeting the whānau (family) and welcoming them. From there I enquire if the person I'm meeting with or

DOI: 10.4324/9781003187042-9

someone in their whānau would like to do a karakia or customary blessing for us. If they are not confident or sure, I let them know that I'm happy to do it. We then move on to whanaungatanga. This is a round of introductions in which they are invited to share who they are: their places of belonging, such as their maunga (mountain) and awa (river); any tribal affiliations they may have; other family connections and any other details they wish to share. If they are not sure, I may prompt them by asking questions such as, 'Where are you from? Where do you live? Where are your whānau from?' If there are some details they don't mention which I'm curious about, I may ask further questions for clarification. For example, 'Have you got any favourite aunties or uncles you go to when you have a problem on your mind?'

One of the first things I think of is to find some way to whakamana (acknowledge the mana or authority of) the person and their whānau. I am aiming for a more level playing field. I am always interested to know about things they are good at, that help them feel confident. For example, perhaps they sing, play the guitar or enjoy kapa haka (Māori cultural performance). When I find out about that, I will spend some time understanding what they are passionate about.

Next, we get on to what brought them to see me. I may ask, 'How do you think I might be able to help you?' During this part of the enquiry, I am conscious that the people I meet are often very respectful of my age and status as an elder. However, I make it clear to those present that I don't consider myself an expert. I want to give respect back to them. They are the ones who know their experience and know what kind of help they are seeking. The purpose of my approach here is to make their kaupapa (purpose) the centre of what we are focusing on.

As I mentioned before, my kuia (female elder) always spoke of the importance of whakaiti: 'always be the least of the least.' Egan also referred to this in Chapter 5; it is better that the kūmara (sweet potato) does not speak of its own sweetness. On the one hand, this was considered good etiquette in my whānau: it was just the right way to behave. On the other hand, my kuia wanted us to remain under the spiritual radar. This is about keeping ourselves safe spiritually. People who come into my space carry things with them. For example, if I truly believe that we are spiritual beings, then it follows that each person I meet carries a whole whakapapa (genealogical) line with them. I would assume that their tīpuna (ancestors) may be present in the room with us. If they see a haughty, loud and proud Tūhoe boy, it may be the unseen ones who take exception to my manner. It is possible that they might decide to teach me a lesson. I have had enough of that kind of learning experience that I prefer to remain humble as much as I can: not just in sessions but in all areas of my life.

As I enquire about the matters that have brought them along, they may talk about spiritual, mental, physical, and family questions, problems, or distress. Frequently, people consult me with experiences that have been puzzling for them. As I explained in Chapter 1, I am interested in the details of their experiences. If they are seeing figures or hearing voices or other sounds, I am curious to know more about what they notice. How many voices are there? Do they recognise the tone of the voice or the appearance of any apparition they are seeing? Does the voice sound male or female? What time of day do they hear or see them?

Once I have that picture, then I am considering what I call a process of elimination to help me discern the cause of their experiences. There is a question, 'He aha te pūtake?' (What is the root cause? What is the origin of what is going on for this person?). I carefully consider if this young person with distressing or unusual experiences may be matekite (spiritually aware). I listen to the details they describe and use my own awareness to discern if this might be the case. I may also ask, 'Have you had these kinds of experiences earlier in your life?' 'Are there other whānau members who have had similar experiences?' 'Is there any known matekite in your family?' 'Have you got any tohunga (Māori healers) you know of in your whakapapa line?' If they give positive responses to any of these questions, this could support a hypothesis that they might be matekite.

Even if I conclude that they are having matekite experiences, if those experiences are distressing, I will consider the following possibilities in my process of elimination. Is there anything in their life or in their past that may be contributing to opening up kūaha to unpleasant perceptual experiences like voices or visions? I'm interested to know if they are using any tarutaru (cannabis) or other drugs. Have they been subject to any trauma in their life that may be significant, such as emotional, physical or sexual abuse? Have they had a traumatic brain injury or other physical trauma? All these factors could alter someone's mind. They could render them vulnerable to negative spiritual entities and experiences. But it doesn't only come from this lifetime. I am also interested in pūtake (root causes) that may come from the generations before. Sometimes the answer lies in transgressions from our forefathers and foremothers that have not been resolved, where there hasn't been any restoration, reparation or reconciliation. I am interested to enquire as far back as seven generations or more.

Explaining Matekite

If I conclude that the person in front of me is having matekite experiences, then, having explained my conclusion, I take time to kōrero (speak) to them and their whānau about the meaning of matekite, as I explained in Chapter 1. Then, I tell the whānau that the best way of helping this young person is to support them, to embrace the situation, to awhi that person in order for them to understand and feel confident that they are not mentally unwell. If these gifts are known in the whānau, then they may well have knowledge about how to look after them. They will already understand that the best strategy is to whakamana them. I would always acknowledge the whānau for their awareness of awhi, manaaki and tiaki – embracing, supporting and protecting the person while they learn about their ability and how to live with it.

In supporting the person, I may kōrero with the whānau about how best to offer a listening ear. Ngāwari is an attitude of patience and going with the flow. It's about gentle enquiry, taking the time they need and not jumping to conclusions. It's all tied up with aroha (love). It's about giving them the mana (spiritual authority) to begin, continue and finish the kōrero when they decide. It may involve putting aside your many roles as a pakeke (adult) in a young person's life and humbly inviting them to kōrero. If they are seeing or hearing things, they may say something that you don't expect. Take the time to understand what they are trying to express. One of the reasons why some young people remain silent is because adults in their life have told them, 'Don't be stupid!'

I like to assist the whānau to identify someone the person can go to who best understands their experiences to help them figure out puzzling perceptions and ensure they are listened to. It's important to kōrero about it in the whānau, so it's not silenced. We discuss a shared language they can use so that the young person has some words to assist them in communicating their experiences. For example, when they see someone standing in the corner, they may wish to refer to their experience as seeing a kēhua, or an apparition. I may talk about some ways in which they may have become more vulnerable to negative spiritual entities. The only problem with that language is that people may find it hard to imagine what an entity is. Therefore, I often refer to such entities as gremlins, clingons or ngāngara (insects or creepy-crawlies). For example, if people are aware of the *Gremlins* movie from the 1980s, gremlins could be mischievous, ugly, silly and sometimes a bit nasty. In order to explain what a clingon is, I use the example of somebody stepping out of their shoes with sweaty feet. If I put my feet in their shoes I will pick up the residue of their sweat. A clingon is like that. If somebody has that spiritual baggage with them and I put on their coat, or put on a taonga (precious pendant) that belongs to them, I may inadvertently take on the clingons they carry with them. My purpose here is to help people understand that such entities are outside of them and they don't have to accept them. No negative entity has power over you unless you allow it. It is possible to exercise your mana, your authority, and those things will have to leave.

I may use a pūrākau (narrative) relating to my own life experience to further explain the nature of matekite. For instance, I sometimes tell people about my earliest experiences of seeing and hearing things others couldn't see and hear, when I was three years old. I tell how my kuia understood what was happening to me and would guide me.

I often talk about the veil of death. When someone dies, it can seem like they have gone out of our lives permanently. However, from a wairua point of view, they have just passed beyond that thin curtain or veil of death. Some people have the ability to see through that veil and catch glimpses of those who are on the other side. At the time of death, the body and the brain may perish, but the mind lives on.

I view matekite as a taonga (precious inherited gift). I take it for granted that we are spiritual beings and we have been put here in this life for a purpose. If you have the ability to see the unseen, then I maintain that your gift has been provided to you in order that you might help someone else. Most people I meet have come through difficult experiences in their lives. I encourage them to consider how they can use the knowledge they may have gained from those hard times to contribute to the lives of others.

Matekite experiences can be in each of the five physical sense modalities: seeing, hearing, tasting, smelling and touching. But there are more: for example, feeling a presence of someone or something in the space around you and feeling a sensation inside your body. Then there is intuitive knowing which I call 'rongo'. For instance, knowing when a situation feels wrong. Or having a strong feeling that you're going to get hurt when there is no other logical reason to think so. That could be 'knowing'. Tairongo is a word that refers to all those senses. It's the whole lot lumped together. Each person with matekite will have their own unique package of sensory abilities.

Tuning In

Quite often people who are seeing visions and hearing voices have been advised by those around them to ignore their perceptions. For those with wairua experiences who are not majorly distressed by them, I often advise the opposite.

Titiro means to look. But it can also mean to observe. I encourage those who are tuned in to wairua but have been afraid of it to begin to explore their gift. To learn about it by sitting quietly and just noticing. Observing what might emerge when they listen to the silence, or sitting watchfully when at first it appears that there is nothing there to see.

Here is an example of how tuning in to wairua can give unexpected information. This kōrero comes from an interaction between my wife, Lesley, Allister and me. Lesley is a wairua practitioner and wairua practitioner trainer. At the time of writing, she was a trainer at a Māori health provider in South Auckland, where I was also working. Allister was asking us about the difference between seeing with our physical eyes and seeing spiritually. After Lesley answers this question, Allister asks her to describe a recent instance.

Lesley: It's a kind of seeing. There's a seeing like most people see with their physical eyes when someone is physically present. And then there's a spiritual perception. You can't see it physically, but it's a certain kind of seeing. I don't know how to explain it.

Allister: So, is it okay if I ask you for an example? The other day when you felt like your friend's ancestor was there, what was your experience?

Lesley: It was their grandmother.

Allister: How did you know it was their grandmother?

Lesley: I didn't see with my eyeballs, but I just knew there was a female presence there. There's a different feeling, masculine and feminine. And the more I focused my inside on her, the clearer it got.

Allister: What was clear though? Was it like a visual image? Or did it feel like someone was present near you, in space?

Lesley: I saw something blue. In my mind's eye, there was a flash of blue. But I knew it was a blue that goes on top of your head with a white border. I didn't see her face. I just knew she was a she. And the feeling I had about time was interesting. I could tell it wasn't in the present time.

Allister: Hmm.

Lesley: If I had a little more time, maybe I could have sat and focused on that. But we were in the middle of a class and my friend was at the edge of my table, so I was needing to listen to the teacher and not look. I could feel it was female, and not male without looking there. It's an inside looking.

Allister: An inside looking?

Wiremu: You know when it's somebody who's close. You can feel it. If you sense somebody is there and you can feel that grandchild-grandmother thing … there's that loving tenderness …

Lesley: Thank you. The feminine aspect of it was that love. It didn't feel like it was someone who was still here. So it wasn't someone who was still alive.

Allister: You said you could feel the time?

Lesley: Yeah. It didn't feel here and now. It felt older. And so I focused on whereabouts in time. I don't know how to put that into words either. It didn't feel like my friend's mother, who I know. But it felt like it was on their father's side. And so I felt into that more. And it didn't feel like their father's time. It felt older. So, I don't know for sure if it was their grandmother. However, my instinct was that it was their father's mother.

Wiremu: And it didn't feel threatening or anything, eh?

Lesley: It felt like love. So that's what made it feel female.
Allister: Hmm. Why?
Wiremu: Why can't males feel loving?
Lesley: It's a different feeling for me than when I feel a masculine presence. It doesn't mean that it feels like that to everybody. But to me, that's how female feels. When I told my friend what I felt, they showed me a picture of their grandmother. When I looked at it carefully, there wasn't anything there that went 'Yes! That's it!' So, my sense about who she was didn't come from seeing the photo. It was based purely on those feelings. She felt like she was from an older time, but in a younger mode – like she was in her 20s or 30s.

Wiremu teaches our spiritually sensitive people to keep a journal of their experiences so that they can learn more about their own subtle perceptions. So, if you are aware of a sensation in your body, and it seems to be related to, for example, a person who has experienced violence in their life, then next time you feel the same sensations you can write it down in your journal. And if you record, for example, five instances, and each time your experience feels similar, you can begin to trust those sensations as a reliable guide. And so for me, I've come to know that particular feeling of 'feminine' over time.
Wiremu: You can then start to develop accuracy …
Lesley: This feminine feeling had a softness. It felt like flannelette pyjamas to me. It felt like comfort and gentleness. Like love wrapping you up. But I've also felt other types of female presence: for example, a 'no muck around' rangatira or matriarch feeling. Like I'm in the presence of a powerful and purposeful leader. At other times I've experienced a staunch warrior type of female energy. So it's not like I don't have other experiences of feminine energy.

Lesley is describing how she was able to sit with an experience even when she was distracted by another activity. By focusing on these subtle aspects of her experience, Lesley was able to open that perceptual doorway just a little.

One way that I explain matekite relates to the word 'kūaha'. From one point of view this means door or entranceway. However, if we enquire more deeply, 'kū' is an inarticulate sound, and 'te hā' refers to the breath. Therefore, 'te kū-a-hā' could be understood as the sound of the breath. In te ao Māori (the Māori world), there is the belief that the Creator breathed into our nostrils, and we became living beings. The top of the nose is closely related to a place between the physical eyes that some cultures refer to as the third eye. This is often understood as relating to the gift of seeing or perceiving things spiritually. I believe that when the Creator breathed into our nostrils, we were given not only life but also the possibility of a doorway to the spiritual realm. But this is an entranceway that we need to be careful with. If we open that door, we may inadvertently welcome in things that we don't understand: entities that are beyond our comprehension. Whatever is there, once it is able to come through, it may be able to alter the way we behave. It may have positive or negative effects on our wellbeing. This is why I emphasise caution. Soon we will talk about some states that can open up these doorways in problematic ways. But first I want to describe concepts in te ao Māori that shed light on people going silent in response to hearing voices or seeing visions.

Noho Puku

If something happened to me such as seeing an apparition or kēhua standing in the corner, rather than tell you about it, I may just sit on it. That's the literal meaning of noho puku. I am holding my experience inside and keeping it to myself. Noho puku could be a positive or negative state. For example: keeping things to myself, thinking about it before I tell others, may be a wise course of action. Some people speak about experiences before they think them through, which can result in judgemental responses from others who don't understand.

The negative side of noho puku can be viewed as an unseen consequence of colonisation. After the time that Western medical practices became dominant, people had to keep their spiritual experiences inside themselves in order to avoid being misdiagnosed by psychiatrists and treated inappropriately. For example, in the decades after the Tohunga Suppression Act (1907), the expression 'mate Māori' came into common usage. I don't use that expression anymore because now it's well known that there is a spiritual realm and sometimes we're affected by things from that world. 'Mate Māori' means 'Māori sickness', and it was used as a way to interact with the medical system, to label something that doctors couldn't understand. Mate Māori is just another way of referring to people being negatively affected spiritually. Since the 1980s, I've hardly heard it used. We don't have to use that term now because we can talk about spiritual distress. We've learnt that people have similar experiences all around the world.

Kuhu

If I am well in myself and supported by whānau and others in my life, and if my mana, mauri (life force) and tapu (sacredness) are in a good space, then I may be able to use internal resources to understand what is happening to me. 'Kuhu' is to go inside to work something out. There is a saying,

'Me kuhu koe i a koe tonu,' which means, 'One should go into oneself to look for the answers.' When people go to church and pray, they commonly put their eyes upward or downward. We often look for an outside source when we could be looking inward. I maintain that divinity is within us. If we are spiritual beings experiencing a human existence, then one purpose in life can be to find out who we really are and what power we hold at our fingertips.

Alongside this, I believe we are divinely connected to the universe and to nature. Having faith in these connections can be protective. I try to be careful not to impose what I believe on anyone else. Any person I meet, I respect their faith and their Source. When people are searching, a starting point for me is encouraging them to consider that they have the mana, the authority to heal themselves and determine their own Source.

Kahupō

In Chapter 2 I told the narrative of Rūaumoko, the youngest of all the children of Papatūānuku (Mother Earth) and Ranginui (Sky Father), who was trapped inside his mother after his parents had been separated by Tāne. There, cloaked in darkness in his waikahu or amniotic fluid, over time he felt alienated and confused. He was unable to see anything. He couldn't see where he was, nor could he see any pathway forward. This state of confusion, ignorance and fear is what I refer to as kahupō. Such a state could come about if a person is matekite and suffering from negative spiritual experiences that they don't understand and they have no one to help guide them. It could also come about for someone who is matekite and using cannabis, and their supernatural doorways get jammed open. In this situation, they could experience kahupō and this may start to resemble what psychiatrists may refer to as a psychotic state.

Kahupō can happen when a person is withholding their experience from the scrutiny of others: from a fear of not being believed or being ridiculed. They can start questioning their sanity. For many people, that anxiety about whether they may be losing their mind is hugely stressful. For some, this feeling of isolation and being estranged from family and friends can contribute to a state of whakamomori. At this point, a person's turmoil has reached such an intensity that they may consider doing something desperate. They may yearn for a simple way out of their predicament, sometimes resulting in suicide.

Environment

There are certain conditions that I believe can contribute to young people who are spiritually aware becoming more vulnerable to negative spiritual entities, which can lead to distressing voices and visions. Some of these are environmental factors that may be present on and off in their life and may have a low-level contribution that only becomes a big problem later, at a crisis point. Here are a few examples which might seem minor and commonplace to some people.

When we allow our tamariki (children) to watch horror movies, we can inadvertently contribute to opening up their spiritual doorways, rendering them vulnerable to uninvited negative entities. The same applies to young people who are permitted to watch pornography. When kids spend a lot of time playing first-person shooter video games – watching how to kill people, the best way to sneak around, when to pull the trigger – these experiences are mind-altering. Through so many repetitions, these patterns start to affect their psyche. A sensitive young person is more likely to be affected like this, especially if they have experienced family violence or sexual abuse and may be fantasising about a way to punish the perpetrator. Such experiences are harmful emotionally and psychologically. However, I maintain the spiritual impact is even more significant. These mind-altering experiences can lead to a young person being less protected from negative spiritual energies.

Trauma

For people who have had traumatic experiences such as family violence or sexual abuse, I often talk about the impact of these experiences on their mana, mauri and tapu (NiaNia et al., 2017a, 2017b).

We all possess mana due to the divine connection to our Source. We are sacred beings. It is possible for that sacredness, that tapu, to be violated by an act such as physical, emotional or sexual abuse. When that happens, the affected person may feel like they have lost some of their mana. Some people try to get their mana back through various means, such as using drugs or through sex or gambling. Others might seek mana by climbing the corporate ladder or owning the biggest car. However, seeking mana outside of us is fruitless. Ultimately, we all possess that mana; it is never lost. When your tapu has been violated, it can feel like you have been broken. This could negatively affect your mauri or life force. It is still there but may be diminished due to that trauma.

In addition, there are other ways that trauma can affect people, even before they have conscious memory. There is a text that says, 'Out of the belly shall flow rivers of living water.' When you were in your mother's womb, what was her environment like? How was she treated by those around her? If she was subject to violence or verbal abuse, for example by her partner, her unborn pēpē (baby) can be affected. The pēpē is encased in the amniotic sac, filled with living water. I believe that water has memory, and this can contribute to negative spiritual impacts on this pēpē, as well as the physiological effects of stress hormones and other factors.

But not only this: we are all standing in a stream of wairua that comes down to us from our ancestors. When your mother gave birth to you, the amniotic sac broke, and out of that water came you. When your mother's mother gave birth to her, she emerged out of that water. If there has been pollution or contamination in the form of trauma and other difficulties upstream, then it could come down and affect you. I believe that it is possible to address the intergenerational trauma that is impacting the wairua of a person and their whānau. In doing so, the spiritual doorway that has been jammed open by this trauma can be closed and disturbing voices and visions can become much more manageable. I maintain that it's not just DNA, epigenetics and behaviour that we inherit from our parents; wairua can be just as important and sometimes more so.

Tarutaru

Drugs are a major problem for many people, let alone those who are matekite. Often distressed young people seek comfort from drugs. Those who are spiritually aware are much more vulnerable to substances like cannabis opening up a supernatural doorway that they are not prepared for. In Chapter 5, Egan described the initial relief he felt from cannabis and how this lured him into using more and more. This paradoxical effect of cannabis is not well recognised and people may assume that smoking is helping them. However, the opposite often occurs. In those situations, the person's spiritual doorways can get jammed wide open. It may be very hard to close them, and all kinds of rubbish from the other side can pour through. At times like this, if things get extreme, then young people may develop a psychotic illness. If they have a purely spiritual problem, I would be confident that karakia could be helpful to address that. With drug-induced experiences which may be psychosis, my first advice would be: 'Stop smoking dope.' A karakia is not a quick fix for cannabis-related voices and visions. Even though I would still view the problem as a spiritual one, before anything further can be done, you need to stop using whatever is jamming the doorway open.

Some Indigenous cultures have used cannabis and hallucinogens to facilitate contact with the spiritual world. Generally, however, training and practices to guide those who are being initiated into its use have been handed down over many generations to protect them from being overwhelmed. People who are using cannabis and other drugs recreationally and are vulnerable in other ways to negative spiritual experiences are putting themselves at risk. For anyone who is matekite, I would recommend avoiding cannabis and other substances entirely.

Role of Whānau

I have already described the powerful role that whānau can have in supporting the wellbeing of their whānau members. This is particularly illustrated in Chapter 5, with Egan's whānau having such an important healing role in his life. Likewise, Grace in Chapter 7 gained similar benefit from the patience, understanding, love and guidance from her mother and other whānau members.

However, there is one different matter that I wish to comment on here. Sometimes, when tamariki or rangatahi (young people) are experiencing visions and hearing voices, the whānau decide that a good solution is to ask a tohunga to shut down their gift. The logic of shutting down someone's matekite is that hopefully they won't continue to see or experience things that might put them at risk of developing mental health problems. Perhaps that comes about because elsewhere in their whakapapa there were others with similar gifts that were misunderstood or associated with mental health problems; for example, due to the use of tarutaru or other drugs. I've never helped shut someone's matekite down. My view is that it is a gift. For the wellbeing of the person and their whānau, it's best to let it have a natural run. However, if people are having negative experiences, then I am looking to identify the pūtake. If they are using substances, then we need to address that. If there is mamae, pain from the past, that may well be contributing to their spiritual predicament. Once it has been possible to address the abuse they've been through, whether that be psychologically, physically or spiritually, then healing to me would involve giving manaaki to that person to help them embrace their matekite.

A further matter relates to the use of psychiatric medication. There are situations when someone is experiencing a lot of negative spiritual experiences but it looks to the whānau and the mental health team like they are suffering from a psychotic illness. Often, they would be prescribed psychiatric medication such as antipsychotic drugs. In this situation, sometimes the medication may have some effect in shutting down the person's experiences. However, for some of us antipsychotic medication may have the opposite effect. Egan's situation from Chapter 5 is a good illustration of that. I also accept that there are some situations, such as severe depression or psychosis, when psychiatric medication can have a beneficial effect. My reservation about such treatments is that while they may sustain the person at that difficult time, they do not heal the person or cure the problem. They provide a temporary solution. From my perspective, unless you are able to find the root cause and address that, unless there is healing, it may be very unclear when the person is able to cease taking such treatment and remain well.

There is a saying, 'Kimihia te pūtake kia kitea he huarahi' (Search for the source of the problem, and there you may find healing). Such a process will need to be at the right pace for the person I'm meeting with. There needs to be a spirit of partnership. For me, the purpose is healing.

10 Huakina

Wiremu NiaNia, Allister Bush, and Caleb

Wiremu

Throughout this book, we have opened doorways to Māori and psychiatric knowledge about the meanings of voices and visions. This final chapter is about the application of these ideas to clinical practice in mental health.

Te Hua means 'the fruit' and the word huakina means 'to open'. This chapter is focused on the fruit of all the kōrero (explanation) from previous chapters. We believe that sharing such knowledge is only of value if that information is applied properly. Huakina implies multiple openings and there are many possible approaches to explore whether people might be having wairua (spiritual) experiences when they are hearing voices or seeing visions. We are not saying these ideas are the only way.

I hand over to Allister to start this kōrero from his clinical perspective, and I add my own whakaaro (views) in response.

Allister

I do not consider myself an expert in Māori mental health or people's experiences of wairua. However, I accept Wiremu's view that those of us who are clinicians have a responsibility to educate ourselves to a sufficient level about how to recognise patterns that might indicate that a person may be having Māori spiritual experiences as part of what is going on for them.

As a psychiatrist, I'm interested in how clinicians can assist people to figure out whether their voices and visions are spiritual experiences or symptoms of a psychiatric problem. If they are having spiritual experiences, they may benefit from seeing a Māori healer, wairua practitioner or other Māori expert such as a kaumātua (elder), as well as their mental health clinician. If they are having hallucinations and other psychotic phenomena rather than spiritual experiences, they can be offered appropriate mental

DOI: 10.4324/9781003187042-10

health care and treatment. In other situations, for example, if someone is experiencing both psychotic symptoms and spiritual voices and visions together, a combination of approaches may be appropriate.

I agree with Wiremu that Māori healing expertise should be freely available to anyone needing it. However, Māori healing is not yet recognised as an accepted discipline in mainstream mental health services in Aotearoa (NiaNia et al., 2017b). As a result, Māori practitioners with relevant expertise may not be easy to access.

Consultation with kaumātua and other Māori experts is the most appropriate way to discern whether the person and their whānau (family) might benefit from a consultation with a Māori healer. To assist clinicians, we return to some of the practical approaches we suggested in our first book to help determine whether a person is having wairua experiences or psychiatric symptoms or both (NiaNia et al., 2017b). We explore these approaches through the experiences of several young people and offer some key questions to ask.

Exploring Experiences

I had known Kevin, aged 14, for several years and had been seeing him for regular therapy as his psychiatrist for some months when one day he arrived at our session, sat down and recounted an unusual experience from lunchtime at his school several days before.

Kevin: I saw this Māori lady from the past; she was wearing a really nice cloak-type thing. And she was talking to me. I couldn't understand a word of it.

Allister: Do you think she was talking to you in te reo Māori (the Māori language)?

Kevin: Mmm. She was. But then she reached out and grabbed my hand. I was sitting on the [school] field. And all I could see was trees. Trees, trees, trees, risen up from the ground. There was nothing around. Even all the buildings were gone.

Kevin then explained that the woman had taken him to what he thought was the local marae (ceremonial meeting house), but in an older time.

Allister: So you are still sitting in the same spot … on the grass?

Kevin: Yeah. But it's like my spirit went to there.

Allister: Because where you are at [school] you normally wouldn't be able to see [the marae] at all. How did you know it was that marae?

Kevin: It felt like it was there. It was a small settlement though. It wasn't as large as it is today.

Allister: What could you see there?
Kevin: It was like wooden fences ... stuck up like thatching. They were pretty high. The marae ... it was a beautiful design ...
Allister: Were you seeing it in colour or black and white?
Kevin: Colour. The wood they made it out of was that, I don't know the name for it, but it was that really strong red wood.

In response to my questions, Kevin recounted that at the marae he could see people walking around and saw some men carrying taiaha (long wooden Māori weapons). He continued, 'They didn't look hostile. They just kept walking. They didn't seem to notice me.' He explained that the woman continued to speak in te reo throughout the experience and spoke no English at all. He felt like she was asking him who he was. He emphasised he was trying to explain to her, 'I don't understand te reo. I'm trying to learn.'

Kevin: It finished by her running back with me. Like ... we ran back to the trees. I didn't run.
Allister: You weren't physically running?
Kevin: I wasn't physically running ... yeah. But we were running through the bush. And then, I just fell to the ground. And then came back to reality.

Kevin told me that during this lunchtime he had been sitting on the grass at school by himself. Having had his lunch, he had been feeling okay. 'If anything, I was feeling rather bored.' When I asked him to describe more of his experience of her cloak, he said, 'It not only looked but felt special. When she was right in front of me, I reached out to touch it and the feathers felt very soft. They were not just ordinary feathers.'

The woman looked young, perhaps in her late 20s, and Kevin was puzzled about why she would seek him out, given that he wasn't from the local iwi. He assumed she was from the local iwi and from an earlier time. When I asked him about how she treated him, he responded, 'She was really nice. She didn't act real staunch or really scary. She was, like, real kind. She wasn't there to hurt me.' He estimated that the experience had gone on for as long as ten minutes. He said, 'I don't know what to think about this experience. I've never had one like it before. It freaked me out a little. But new things normally freak me out. I guess it was probably a spiritual experience.'

Wiremu has already outlined his practice for addressing Māori protocols in a consultation in Chapter 9. What follows are a few principles for engaging with Māori individuals and whānau, outlined for non-Māori readers and clinicians unfamiliar with Māori settings.

Māori Matters to Consider

Manaaki

Wiremu has explained the importance of manaaki, such as practices of hospitality that acknowledge the mana (spiritual authority) of the other person. For Māori whānau and clinicians, this won't need any emphasis. Having worked at Te Whare Mārie for many years, I am now more familiar with such practices, but in my early years at our service, due to my mainstream medical training, I was slow to understand their significance in building rapport with Māori young people and their families.

Kevin had been working with our cultural therapist, Rongo Larkin, over the previous year. Rongo has worked at Te Whare Mārie on and off since the early 1990s, and practices of manaaki are integral to his manner of interacting with young people and their whānau members. His manner of warmly greeting the whānau, acknowledging whakapapa (genealogy) connections, encouraging individuals to be in the driving seat of decisions about their care, and building up young people in the words he uses are deeply embedded in his practice. On a number of occasions when Kevin had been suspended from school, Rongo turned up to support him and to facilitate problem-solving meetings with his teachers and whānau. He always had encouraging words to sustain Kevin in his low points and help maintain his self-respect and sense of agency.

Tikanga

The significance of tikanga (Māori protocol) will also be apparent to Māori readers but may not be to Pākehā (New Zealand European) readers and clinicians unfamiliar with Māori settings. Kevin had grown up with more contact with the Pākehā side of his family and often had feelings of alienation towards his Māori ancestry. Rongo introduced Kevin to the use of karakia (prayers) and taught him karakia that came from Kevin's ancestral area. He fostered Kevin's use of the te reo he was learning at school and supported him to strengthen his ties to his Māori whānau. During our therapy sessions, Kevin would open and close our sessions with his karakia. Even though Kevin had previously felt strongly inclined to reject his Māori identity, this was no longer the case. Rongo also involved Kevin in events on our marae such as pōwhiri (ceremonial welcome) and included him in food preparation and other activities in our wharekai (dining hall).

There are many ways for Pākehā and other clinicians to become more familiar with tikanga and te reo. For example, the Takarangi Competency Framework (Matua Raki, 2009) is a structured learning model that supports clinicians to further develop a wide range of Māori competencies within their own clinical context.

Whānau

Seeing someone in their relational context is often a helpful way of enhancing exploration of possible wairua meanings relating to their experiences. Kevin, at this time, was unenthusiastic about involving his family directly in sessions. However, five years earlier, when he had been in frequent trouble at school, Kevin reported seeing an old lady in his classroom that no one else could see. She told him her name and said, 'Everything will be okay.' Despite this, he was upset about seeing her as he didn't know what to make of it.

We subsequently met with Kevin and his caregivers, his Pākehā grandparents. Kevin had not told them about this experience, perhaps because he felt anxious that they might disapprove. However, once he was persuaded to share this incident with them, his grandmother became tearful and revealed that the name the old lady had given Kevin was the name of her own deceased mother. She said the woman he described sounded very similar to his great-grandmother, even though Kevin had never met her. She concluded Kevin was capable of having spiritual experiences and revealed that other members of her family had also had such experiences.

Tātaihono

In Wiremu's description of tātaihono in Chapter 1, he referred to binding the Māori and Pākehā elements together in a way that enhances the mana of both Māori healing and psychiatry. I find this idea intriguing because I would usually associate binding something with constraining it in some way. But here Wiremu is suggesting quite the opposite. In addition, he is proposing that neither of us need to compromise the assumptions and values that form the basis of our respective knowledge systems.

We each have our own knowledge bases. Wiremu has expertise in wairuatanga (spirituality), Māori healing, Māori language, tikanga and other aspects of Māori knowledge. My discipline relates to medical and psychiatric theory and practice. The mutual respect that Wiremu talks about is enacted in a historical context in which Māori knowledge has been most often silenced or ignored in medical and psychiatric settings in our country. Therefore, I see part of my role as educating myself about how these silencing processes have occurred and playing an active role in highlighting that and creating space for Wiremu to articulate his understandings. I am often curious about Wiremu's point of view and will invite him to clarify aspects of it. However, my curiosity needs to be tempered with an awareness that I am certainly capable of being overbearing in my questions. While he is very patient with me, I need to be aware of that balance.

Wiremu has said that one thing that matters to him is that we were able to start out with a level playing field. I think that Wiremu was being extremely generous to suggest it was level. I don't see it that way. When we first worked together, the medical hierarchy was present even at our Māori mental health service. While Māori worldviews were strongly valued, Māori healing knowledge was an insubstantial part of the discourse in team meetings. So that didn't seem to be a level playing field.

In another way, I don't feel it is a level playing field even now. I consider myself to have a junior role in this partnership. When we are meeting with a family together, my view is that they are there to meet Wiremu and benefit from his knowledge and approach. It's my role as a psychiatrist to support that and to make it clear to the family that I value what he has to say alongside any psychiatric perspective I might have. I consider him to have status as an elder. It is my job to support him in that role and endeavour to take care of various practices of hospitality, whether that be fetching him a cup of tea, arranging transport to an appointment, or making sure his other needs are catered for when we are together. I have tried to learn about how to be around elders from observing other colleagues, such as Rongo Larkin, and his approach to manaaki of kaumātua as well as everyone he comes into contact with.

I see our partnership as a field or space where we are sitting together and relating. In this field, the central relationships are with each other and with the person and family we are meeting with. The partnership between healer and psychiatrist or other clinician comes about through our ability to sit, share and be actively aware of our respective understandings and differences. I see it as important that we each hold on to the knowledge we carry from our own area of expertise. However, I need to hold mine lightly enough to leave plenty of space for listening to Wiremu's point of view. I have always felt heard by Wiremu.

It's also important that we have been in such conversations for many years. There are concepts that Wiremu attempted to explain to me years ago that I didn't grasp at the time. The meaning may suddenly appear more clear to me during a new conversation. This raises another matter for me about positioning. No matter how long I work at Te Whare Mārie, my perspective will always be a Pākehā one. Having spent this much time around Wiremu, it's possible that I may start to develop an inflated sense of myself and what I know about Māori concepts. No matter how much my Māori colleagues remind me that I am 'part of the whānau' at Te Whare Mārie, my viewpoint remains Pākehā. As Egan said in Chapter 5, a little knowledge can sometimes be a dangerous thing. I have frequently made mistakes assuming I understood a Māori concept but later realised there was an important nuance I had missed. One glaring example in writing this book was that I initially disapproved of Wiremu's focus in Chapter 2 on the source of his knowledge coming primarily from his kuia (grandmother), when the usual Pākehā academic style is to focus on written sources.

Of course, Wiremu maintained his position on this, and over time I realised he was right, but I did not have the inherited understanding that a Māori colleague may have had. Understandably, in this partnership, we don't share the same views all the time. I have learnt most from our conversations when I have made the effort to suspend my judgements about what Wiremu has said and to enquire further.

Another example of recognising my Pākehā viewpoint was when someone likened my sense of being a junior partner in this tātaihono partnership to having a tuakana-teina relationship with Wiremu. This refers to an important Māori relationship between siblings of the same gender: tuakana, the elder sibling, and teina, the younger sibling. My response to this suggestion was to realise that I have no idea if the relationship is similar. Even though I have an intellectual understanding of what these concepts mean, my viewpoint is a Pākehā one. I did not grow up in a Māori relational context that would allow me to know what this relationship feels like: to have a visceral understanding of the nuances of this relational scenario. These reasons lead me to believe that there would be major advantages for Māori young people and families to be able to work with Māori psychiatrists, elders and other clinicians.

Decolonising Practices

Wiremu has referred to tātaihono as being about reparation and reconciliation as well as collaboration and connection. Accordingly, it is necessary that I maintain and refresh my awareness of the history between our cultures. Furthermore, there is a history between our professions that I have become more starkly aware of in the writing of this book, as I have seen vividly the way psychiatry has taken an active role in suppressing and overlooking Māori world views about experiences such as voices and visions. Institutional racism has been rife in psychiatric institutions, as we saw from Egan's harrowing hospital experiences in Chapter 5. I hope there have been positive changes in psychiatric hospital care since that time, but reparation and reconciliation in our partnerships require ongoing vigilance. Active decolonising approaches are needed to address these ongoing problems of racism and coercive practices in our mental health systems (Smith, 2012). For those wishing to understand more about decolonisation, Elkington et al. (2020) have written an insightful and refreshing introduction.

From my Pākehā side in this relationship, in order to maintain a decolonising focus, I have to be vigilant about holding my understanding of historical injustices in mind and considering how these may inform our current interactions. I have frequently made mistakes and stumbled around in a clumsy fashion. Wiremu has hardly ever pointed out my behaviour directly. It's not his job to do so. Part of my role is to stay attentive to these dynamics and to reflect with Pākehā friends and co-workers who also have a commitment to finding decolonising ways of working in partnership with Māori colleagues.

While I was writing this chapter, I received a text from a Pākehā colleague working in a Māori workplace referring me to a radio interview with Māori elder, Haare Williams (Williams, 2022). During this interview, Matua Haare talked about what he called the Five Rs: respect, responsibility, responsiveness, reciprocity and reverence. These words sum up attitudes that have been necessary from my viewpoint in my partnership with Wiremu.

For the first of the Five Rs, respect, my attitude is that I need to demonstrate respect for Wiremu's knowledge, status and wisdom when interacting with him, and also make that respect evident to individuals, families and colleagues who meet with us.

The second R, responsibility, comes with being in this partnership. The onus is on me to create space for Wiremu's point of view to be heard when institutions would very likely shut it down, and to ensure others can benefit from his perspectives. From another point of view, I don't consider that Wiremu has the same responsibility from his side. For example, due to the dominance of psychiatric discourse for many years, I don't think Wiremu needs to understand or accommodate Western psychiatric understandings in the way that I have a responsibility to make myself a student of Māori meanings about spirituality.

The third R, responsiveness, can be about noticing and being prepared to address a wrong, whether that's a misunderstanding between us or a broader historical injustice that impinges on our work together.

Matua Haare goes on to describe the fourth R, reciprocity, as being a necessary value. Receiving a koha (offering) from Wiremu, such as some gem of insight, leads me to reflect on how I might be able to offer something in response.

The fifth and final R is reverence. This one interests me because Wiremu has an irreverent sense of humour, and his understated style might render this value less evident. But there are moments in our interactions or in a consultation with a young person or family when something significant happens: perhaps a moment when the rapport deepens, or the young person has become aware of some new understanding about their life, or Wiremu has raised an unexpected matter that turns out to be of central importance for the family. An attitude of reverence can help me appreciate and make time for the spiritual significance that such moments may have for the young person and their family members.

A further way to foster decolonising practice involves processes of cultural accountability, which I referred to in Chapter 1 (Waldegrave et al., 2003). Such practices can be set up in organisations to promote both gender and cultural accountability. In a bicultural agency, for example, having

Māori and Pākehā groups could allow any matters of concern to be addressed between the groups. This does require a high degree of commitment, vulnerability and trust. In my work at Te Whare Mārie, I am mindful of my lines of both clinical accountability and cultural accountability. In terms of cultural accountability, I consider myself accountable to our kaumātua and team leader. In working with Wiremu, I consider myself culturally accountable to him and to the elders and family members with whom we are working. Even so, I realise that Wiremu's style means that he will be very unlikely to raise a matter directly with me even if I may have transgressed some cultural boundary. I think that the principle of reverence can be important here. Given my growing up in the dominant culture and knowing where my discipline sits in terms of professional hierarchy, I realise I have many blind spots. When I have wondered if I have done something that could have caused offence, I have tried to humbly approach Wiremu, explain my concern and seek his response. Reflecting on those moments now, I see that Matua Haare's reverence seems an appropriate description for my experience of the space between us and the sacredness of the relationship in those moments.

Matike Mai

During the preparation of this chapter, a Pākehā friend accustomed to working in partnerships with Māori colleagues suggested I acquaint myself with Matike Mai (Matike Mai Aotearoa, 2016). This framework offers a pathway for constitutional transformation in Aotearoa. It was prepared following a large series of hui led by Margaret Mutu and Moana Jackson between 2012 and 2015 that focused on what Māori want for a governance structure in our country. Matike Mai is based on two important documents: He Whakaputanga o te Rangatiratanga o Nu Tireni, the 1835 Declaration of Independence of the United Tribes of New Zealand, and the 1840 Te Tiriti o Waitangi, New Zealand's founding document.

Matike Mai advocates for a governance structure with three parts: a tino rangatiratanga (Māori sovereignty) sphere of influence, a kawanatanga (Pākehā governance) sphere and a third sphere called the relational sphere. The tino rangatiratanga sphere is where Māori would make decisions for Māori. The kawanatanga sphere is where the Crown would make decisions for its people. The relational sphere is where the two parties would meet to decide what needed to be decided together. It is expected that each party would exercise their authority in different ways, according to their own tikanga and laws. In this framework it is necessary for each to honour the authority of the other. Matike Mai highlights the importance of such principles as balance and conciliation in the processes that would take place in the relational sphere.

I notice similarities in Matike Mai with what Wiremu and I are working towards in our partnership. In the Māori healing playing field, Wiremu has authority. It is not my role to question his perceptions, interpretations, conclusions or use of tikanga. In the psychiatry part of the playing field, it is my role to use principles I have learnt from my discipline to advise the person and family to the best of my ability about a possible mental health understanding of what may be happening for them. Matike Mai was designed to address a constitutional problem, but if it were applied to our situation it would describe a relational part of the playing field. In this space, we would be able to enquire about each other's point of view, reflect together on the situation the young person and family are facing, and develop a shared understanding together and with the family. Wiremu has suggested that working together in this way can enhance the mana and effectiveness of both approaches. To me, it makes sense that this could happen if interactions in this sphere are characterised by the principles of reparation, reconciliation, collaboration and connection, as well as those of respect, responsibility, responsiveness, reciprocity and reverence.

Interview-Based Practices

In this section I outline potential approaches for clinicians to assist people who have unexpected perceptual experiences to identify whether Māori meanings could be relevant to their experiences. If they are relevant, involving a Māori cultural practitioner could help them make sense of their experiences.

Consider whether their experiences have strong cultural congruence and meaning that make sense from Māori points of view

Kevin's account of his experience on the field at his school contained many compelling cultural details. The woman he described had a distinctly Māori physical appearance and was wearing a feather cloak known as a korowai. She was speaking only in te reo, even though Kevin couldn't understand what she said. In addition, there was the visit to the local marae. All these aspects led me to consult Rongo for his opinion.

Kevin also reported a strong feeling that the woman he could see came from 'another time'. As a psychiatrist, I pondered his description and considered possible mental health explanations, but none seemed satisfactory. The incident appeared to occur when he was under no apparent distress or pressure. Perhaps it could have reflected a moment of reverie or fantasy, or it may have been a sheer product of his imagination. However, he did not describe the incident as if it were under his own control. He had not been consuming substances on the day of this event, or for several weeks before.

There was no obvious evidence that he was suffering from a physical brain problem such as seizures to explain his dramatic experience, although he was not assessed by a paediatrician at this time. It is pertinent that he had no further episodes like this in the following weeks.

While Kevin was telling me his story, he had a calm manner and a matter-of-fact way of speaking. On other occasions he could express himself in a far more dramatic fashion, especially if relaying a situation in which he believed himself to have been unjustly treated. He appeared bemused by what had happened and did not appear to be trying to persuade me about any particular aspect of it. However, he was clear that this experience had a vivid and tangible quality, especially his description of reaching out and touching the korowai. If he was hallucinating, then he was having synchronised auditory, tactile and visual hallucinations. In reflecting on all of this, I became increasingly convinced that there could be a cultural or spiritual explanation for his experiences that day. Rongo believed Kevin could be having wairua experiences which was consistent with what we knew about Kevin being tuned into the spiritual realm. We discussed whether to consult a tohunga (Māori healer) but decided this might not be necessary as Kevin hadn't experienced any distress.

Consider whether the voice or vision could be their ancestor

Here are some questions to consider asking a person when thinking about whether a voice or vision could relate to an ancestor.

- What does the voice or do the voices say? Do they ever say things that are friendly or supportive? Do they remind you of anyone in your family? Does the figure you see remind you of anyone who was important in your life in the past? Do they remind you of anyone who is no longer living?
- Has anyone in your whānau ever suggested the voice might be someone related to you? Has anyone ever suggested that you might have a kaitiaki (spiritual guardian)?

In Chapter 8, Wiremu talked about the role kaitiaki can have in the lives of many people. He explained that young people may find communication from their ancestors confusing and even disturbing if they don't have guidance from elders in their family.

Kevin didn't recognise the woman he saw before him at school, but his grandmother was easily able to identify her as Kevin's great-grandmother.

In Chapter 8, Jake described identifying the voices he was hearing as coming from his ancestors. He could distinguish their voices by the content of what they said. Frequently they had reassured him, but they had also been known to correct him if they disapproved of his choices and behaviour. Whilst in psychiatry it is known that auditory hallucinations due to a psychotic illness can include both positive and negative comments, there are a number of other points in Jake's account that support his interpretation that these voices were his kaitiaki. A relative told Jake he had kaitiaki with him, and suggested who these kaitiaki might be. Jake thought the words spoken by one of the voices sounded like they came from his Koro (grandfather), whom Jake had known when his Koro was alive. These words also reminded Jake of the stories he'd heard about his Koro. Wiremu said he saw that Jake had supportive spiritual entities located just next to him, which was further evidence to support Jake's view.

Consider if the person may be having matekite or matakite experiences

Wiremu has defined matekite (spiritual awareness) and matakite (foresight) in Chapter 9. As a Pākehā clinician without access to these gifts, what questions can I ask in an interview to help me identify whether someone I am meeting with may be having matekite or matakite experiences?

The following questions, or 'doorways of enquiry', are offered tentatively, in the hope that they are useful. I expect there are others who will see things differently and may be able to offer better and more comprehensive interview strategies. Before long, I anticipate Māori research into this area will provide further options.

After the list of questions, Wiremu and I each provide a brief commentary.

Doorways of Enquiry

The questions that follow may be useful for clinicians to assist people to identify whether they may be having spiritual experiences. They are intended not as an inflexible interrogation strategy, but as part of a nuanced approach to a sensitively attuned interview. The questions are organised under three categories: recent experiences, developmental history and family history. Questions about recent experiences are divided up into themes relating to sensory details, shared experiences, knowing, dreams and intuition relating to people and places. For any positive responses, follow-up questions would include asking for examples. The first questions relate to experiences that the person has presented with, and which may be concerning them.

Recent Experiences

- **Sensory**
  - Describe your experience in as much detail as you can. What did you hear? What did you see? What did you feel? Did you notice any taste or smell?

    - If you saw a figure or heard a voice, did you also feel something there to explain it, such as a presence near you?
    - Do you ever see colours around people?

- **Shared experiences**
    - Has anyone else heard the voice you hear or felt a presence near you that helped to explain your experience? Has anyone else seen the figure you saw or felt a presence there that helped to explain your experience?

- **Knowing**
    - Have you ever had an experience of knowing something that you couldn't possibly have known?

- **Dreams**
    - Have you ever had dreams that later seemed to come true in a surprising or uncanny way?

- **Intuition about people and places**
    - Have you ever had a strong feeling about a person, such as a stranger, that you couldn't account for by their words or how they looked? For example, perhaps you saw someone who looked scary or mean, but you had a good feeling about them and felt they were a good person? Or have you ever had a strong feeling that there was something not good about a person, even though you couldn't tell from their outward appearance?
    - Do you ever have feelings about places you visit that are hard to account for based on how that place looks? For example, you might visit a building and it's nicely painted but you get a distinctly bad or uneasy feeling there. Or you might visit a place and feel particularly good there without being sure why. Do you ever have any other intuitive feelings about places that are hard to explain?

Developmental History

- Did you ever have experiences like these when you were younger? How old were you? Please given an example.

Family History

- In many Māori families, spiritual experiences are considered quite normal. Who else in your whānau knows about wairua or spiritual experiences? Who else in your whānau has spiritual experiences? What kind of experiences have they talked about?

- Do you have someone in your whānau you could go to for advice about wairua matters? Who do others in your extended whānau go to for help about spiritual matters?

The first questions in this list under 'recent experiences' may help clarify details about a person's unusual perceptions. In Chapter 1, Wiremu suggested paying attention to such details. In psychiatric terms, this relates to the history of the problem or the details of the phenomena they are describing. The nuances of a person's experience can help us work with them to figure out if there is a pattern that seems to fit with a psychiatric symptom, such as a hallucination. Alternatively, exploration of sensory details may help clarify whether the experience could be spiritual in origin. For example, in Chapter 5, Egan shared his own hard-won observation that psychotic experiences present themselves to him generally in one or perhaps two sensory modalities at the same time, such as auditory and/or visual, or visual and/or olfactory. On the other hand, if he can discern the same entity or experience in more than two sensory modalities, he would conclude it is more likely to be a wairua experience.

The questions under 'shared experiences' ask whether anyone else can sense what the person is seeing or hearing. Wiremu discussed shared experiences in Chapter 1, illustrating them with his shearing shed story. In Chapter 8, both Wiremu and Jake were aware of three entities in Jake's flat and could indicate each entity's individual character and where it was in space. Wiremu was also able to identify their relationship with Jake. When a Māori healer or other wairua practitioner can give such assistance, it can provide spiritual evidence that the person is having wairua experiences and help them make sense of their experience. Sometimes people also talk about a pet that appears to be responding to an unseen entity that they can also perceive.

From a psychiatric perspective, questions relating to a person's earlier life are often referred to as their personal history or developmental history. In Chapter 8, Jake's mother described a situation from Jake's preschool years when the two of them visited the urupā (cemetery) where his great-grandfather was buried. Jake's behaviour there – singing using ancient Māori words he didn't know – was so out of the ordinary that his mother concluded this could have been a sign of his wairua connection to his whakapapa and that place.

A further area to explore is known in psychology and psychiatry as family history. Members of a person's extended family may have had similar spiritual experiences. Asking another family member whether they also had unexplained or spiritual experiences when they were young may invite them to share personal stories they have never spoken of before. These narratives may feel intimate and sacred. Such questioning requires a high degree of rapport and sensitivity, and an atmosphere of reverence.

As Wiremu mentioned in Chapter 9, he often enquires about knowledge of wairua matters in the immediate and extended whānau of the person he is meeting. In Chapter 8, Jake had several whānau members who advised him about his experiences of his kaitiaki and who they might be. Such information can alert me as a clinician to the need to consider unusual perceptual experiences as possibly spiritual, given that spiritual awareness is known in this family. As Wiremu has pointed out, such knowledge can be a source of support and reassurance for people having these experiences. In addition, if there is a history in the family of someone who has been diagnosed with a psychotic illness such as schizophrenia, there may be details about the nature of their experiences that can help us figure out if that person might have been spiritually aware as well as possibly having a psychiatric problem.

Next Wiremu comments on enquiring about dreams.

Wiremu

Allister tells me that asking about dreams that later seem to come true in a surprising or uncanny way, is not the usual way that dreams are understood in psychiatry. However, he has noticed that young people who have a background of other spiritual experiences may give examples of such dreams.

I often take note of what people tell me about their dreams. For those who are matakite, who can see the future, it is commonly accepted in te ao Māori that they may be able to see coming events in their moemoeā (dreams).

When my kuia talked about moemoeā, she was referring to either a dream or vision. She made no distinction between dreams which told her about the future and those that didn't. Similarly, she didn't distinguish between her matakite experiences while awake and those when she was dreaming. Of course, people can have dreams which come true by chance. However, for those who are matakite, some have dreams that can be very accurate. People may report disturbing dreams in which someone close to them appears sick in bed, and then soon after that person develops a terminal illness. We have written elsewhere about a young person who had this kind of dream which came true in a way which she found quite disturbing (NiaNia et al., 2017b). Sometimes the content of the dream may be ordinary and the person may not even mention it to anyone but may later recognise the exact situation in their waking life that they saw in their dream. This is what I believe may be happening for some people when they experience déjà vu.

I don't often have dreams that come true, although that has happened to me. However, my kuia had moemoeā which often proved very accurate. I believe she used the insight she gained from her dreams in her healing work, but she usually kept those matters private. I explained in Chapter 2 that she would have visitations in her dreams of people she knew at the moment just before they passed on. She would cry out, and we would wake up, and before dawn she would get us to pack the truck ready to drive to the tangi. However, the dreams she was most likely to talk about related to horseracing. If she woke in the morning after a dream about a racehorse, she would bundle us into the car and drive to whatever race meeting was happening. Sometimes that was in Wairoa or Gisborne, but other times it was hours away. When we got there, she would identify the horse and jockey that she had seen in her dream and place a large bet on them. Generally, her prediction was correct when she bet on information she got from her dream. Looking back, she never took payment for any healing work she did and never asked for any koha (donation). I guess this was one way she got reimbursed for her mahi (work).

Allister's questions also ask if the person has had intuitive feelings about people. Seventeen-year-old Malia gives a vivid example here of this type of experience.

> I was walking through the supermarket. My auntie was making chicken fettuccine, which is one of my favourite dishes. I was feeling happy about that and skipping through the aisles looking for garlic bread. I skipped past this person without really noticing, but a moment later I had a strange experience. Just as I passed them, I felt like I entered some kind of black hole. This massive feeling overwhelmed me. I stopped right there. All the thoughts in my mind blanked out. I could see glimpses of a guy crying and screaming. I saw flashes of his face in absolute terror, as if something terrible was happening to him. I was flooded with intense emotions that went with those scenes. All I could see was this guy and the background was kind of blurry, but he was really clear. I was freaking out thinking, 'Why am I seeing this?' It wasn't until I turned and saw the man I had just passed, standing there looking at tins of food, that I realised what had happened. It was as if passing him, I had somehow taken in part of him. That wasn't the first time this has happened. The experience is quite familiar to me.

The incident that Malia described here is similar to experiences I have had myself. When she walked past that man standing in the supermarket aisle, it's as if she picked up images and feelings from his wairua. In this case, she walked into the space near him and detected these experiences accidentally, and of course she was shocked by what she saw and felt. When she explained this incident to me, the intensity of her experience suggested to me that she was finely attuned to te ao wairua (the spiritual realm). I could also tell that about her just from being in the room with her. Some of my kōrero with her was focused on helping her understand ways that she could take care of herself when she was experiencing the world in this way.

While this moment was overwhelming for Malia, most people who are in tune with the wairua of others in their environment have much more subtle experiences. Because they are so subtle, often they may dismiss the experience as imagined. Or else they may conclude that it was something they picked up in the non-verbal communication from the person, when actually they detected something from wairua. For me there is a clear difference between what I make from the look of a person and what I can discern about them from wairua.

The next questions ask if the person has had intuitive feelings about places. Just like people, trees, plants and even inanimate objects can have their own mauri (life force). Therefore, it makes sense that buildings and places can have a mauri. There are places that can hold the memory of certain events and a sensitive person may be able to detect that.

In recent years, alongside wairua practitioner training, my wife, Lesley, and I have been running matekite wānanga (spiritual awareness workshops) in which we are helping people who are matekite to understand and further develop such gifts. One of the training activities we include involves the rōpū (group) visiting particular sites, under the guidance of a local kaumātua. At each of these sites events have occurred. These include events of major significance to one of my iwi (tribes). On a site visit, workshop participants are invited to take their time to sit with all of their senses and see what they can pick up. Then we meet back at the training venue and everyone shares what their impressions were. Then our kaumātua tells the story of what is known locally about the events that happened there. On each occasion we find that some of our participants' impressions of the wairua of the place accurately reflect the history of that place. Some workshop participants will progress to wairua practitioner training. In the future, we hope that wairua practitioners can be recognised and employed in the mainstream health workforce alongside other health professionals.

Allister

Diagnostic and Formulation Doorways

Carefully considering diagnostic possibilities when meeting a person describing voices or visions may help clinicians identify situations when these perceptual experiences could be related to spiritual awareness or wairua, or could have some other explanation, including mental illness.

In Jake's situation in Chapter 8, he was hearing voices from time to time. Both he and Wiremu could identify a stimulus for voices that arose outside Jake. Therefore, Wiremu and I agree that they don't qualify as hallucinations according to the DSM-5 definition. However, setting aside the question of whether Jake's experiences had an external stimulus, his voices were vivid, clear and not under voluntary control, and he heard them when he was awake and not under the influence of any substances. As a result, a clinician could view them as consistent with auditory hallucinations.

It is necessary here to consider whether Jake's experiences could have been illusions, products of his imagination, or accounted for by suggestion. Alongside this, did he have any other psychotic symptoms such as disorganised thinking or behaviour, or strongly held false beliefs that would fit with delusions? Other psychotic symptoms such as these would be evidence that might indicate the presence of a psychotic illness. Conversely, the absence of such symptoms in Jake's case could reassure a clinician that his voice-hearing experiences are non-pathological. Given his other matekite experiences, they may be accounted for by his spiritual awareness. The fact that Jake doesn't have any other features of schizophrenia apart from his experience of voices could help a clinician provisionally rule out that diagnosis and offer a culturally informed formulation or shared understanding with Jake and his whānau that accounts for his voices as part of his matekite.

It is not very likely that psychiatrists or other mental health clinicians would mistake Jake's situation for a psychotic illness. However, Egan's illness as an 18-year-old was a more complex scenario. He subsequently described many wairua experiences throughout his earlier life. However, when he was admitted to a psychiatric unit for the first time, it seems likely that he was experiencing not only severe and distressing voices and visions but also beliefs that would qualify as delusions. In addition, his thinking and behaviour were affected negatively to the extent that those around him appear to have been concerned about his wellbeing. I believe most mental health clinicians would conclude that Egan's situation met criteria for a psychotic disorder at the time he was admitted, and they might also consider dissociative voices and visions as a possible explanation in the context of trauma in his life.

If there were major concerns about his safety, such as risk to himself or others, then I believe most if not all mental health clinicians would consider that the safest place for initial treatment would be in hospital. Of course, in Egan's case, I expect he would debate that, due to the harm he experienced while he was there. In retrospect, from Egan's account it is very likely that he was having intense wairua experiences. Would Egan have benefited from a combined psychiatry and Māori healing approach at the time of his first admission? I feel confident that such a partnership would have added a critical extra dimension to his care and his whānau would very likely have embraced such an approach.

A key part of a partnership approach to mental health care can be working with a person and their whānau to develop a shared understanding or formulation of how they came to be in this situation at this time. For Māori, a background of matekite experiences in their early life may be an important factor in such a formulation. This is the case even if they appear to have severe symptoms that are consistent with a psychotic illness. It can help facilitate shared decision-making with the person and their whānau even under the stressful circumstances of such a crisis. A shared formulation can open space for more than one diagnostic conclusion: for example, psychosis, wairua and dissociation as possible explanations for a person's voices or visions. As we saw in Egan's chapter, it could be that each of these explanations accounts for some parts of their experiences. It is possible to hold open two or more differential diagnosis options pending further Māori healing assessment, further psychiatric assessment and discussion between the person, their whānau and the mental health team. Such a formulation could be documented in language acceptable to all parties, or even visually, and could then be added to clinical records and provide a reference point to return to in ongoing planning with the person and their whānau.

The person's description of their experiences can also be documented in ways that create space for cultural as well as psychiatric interpretations. For example, when a clinician is recording mental status examination findings, describing the person's account of their experience in detail, using their words rather than just reducing this to a shorthand label such as 'auditory hallucinations', can facilitate flexible consideration of multiple origins of voices and visions. For a clinician discussing preferred and alternative diagnoses with the person, their whānau and other clinicians, it can be helpful to describe the features that do and don't fit with psychosis, cultural/spiritual phenomena and other explanations, such as trauma. This can illuminate the clinical dilemmas and help the clinician explain, verbally and in writing, the reasoning for reaching their conclusion. It can also demonstrate the clinical logic of further assessment options, such as consulting a Māori healer or treatment options such as antipsychotic medication. Which brings us back to our first point, which is also our final recommendation: the best way to distinguish between Māori spiritual experiences and psychotic symptoms is by consulting with a Māori healer – or wairua practitioner – with appropriate cultural expertise.

A further way to help determine whether a person's experiences of voices and visions are spiritual in nature or relate to a psychiatric problem is to look at the outcome over time. With Jake's story in Chapter 8, he described his ongoing experiences ten years after his original contact with our service. We now return to Caleb's story, which I outlined in Chapter 1, and find out about further developments in his life 14 years after our first meeting.

Catching up with Caleb

As you may recall, Caleb was a 17-year-old Cook Island and New Zealand Māori young man who saw an apparition of a Māori man shouting at him by his letterbox. After our first book was published, Wiremu had blessed a piece of pounamu (greenstone) for Caleb, to thank him for contributing his story. I had contacted Caleb a few times to deliver this to him, but for one reason or another we hadn't been able to meet up. It was now 2021, and the pandemic had been in our lives for more than a year. This time I contacted Caleb, seeking his consent for us to retell his story briefly in Chapter 1. He agreed to meet at a local café.

When we met, Caleb explained that he had been having a very difficult time. Three people he had been very close to had died. The previous year, his beloved grandmother had passed away during the early days of the first New Zealand COVID-19 lockdown. He and his grandfather had nursed her through the final weeks of her life after her long illness. Almost immediately after her death, his grandfather had also been diagnosed with cancer and passed away later that year. A few months later a very close friend died suddenly. He talked about his grief and how hard it had been to pick himself up after losing so many people he loved.

Caleb then asked me about the topic of our current book. When I explained that it was focused on understanding people's experience of voices and visions from Wiremu's Māori healing point of view and my psychiatrist's perspective, his response was, 'That's funny. This morning I had to wake up to make a doctor's appointment before I came out to meet you. My alarm went off, but I rolled over and went back off to sleep. Sometime later I woke up.' In tears now, Caleb explained,

> I was surprised to feel a hand on my chest. Instinctively I knew it was my grandmother. It felt very clearly like she was patting me there, gentle in one way but forcefully enough to wake me, just like she always used to do in the morning. It felt nice. I then distinctly heard her say, 'Rangi.' I would know her voice anywhere. It came from somewhere next to me. And at that moment I realised that I'd slept in and my grandmother was reminding me to ring the doctors. Rangi was the name of our doctor's receptionist. Thinking about it now, I know my grandmother also did this to remind me that she knows what I have been going through: that I have lost pretty much everyone I have been close to.'

He then went on,

> That's not the first time I have heard Nan's voice and known she was there. About a month after my grandfather died, I was living alone, and it happened. I love boiled eggs. My habit is to save time by turning the stove element on high, boiling the jug, putting six eggs in the saucepan and then pouring the boiling water over the top. This time I put them on and went and lay on my bed. I watched a little more of a movie I was watching, but in a short time fell asleep. Suddenly I heard my Nan's voice in a panic calling me, "Bubba, Bubba!" I woke with a start. As I sat up, even though I was in my bedroom, I could see her standing there in her nightie and it looked like she was in the kitchen. She was shaking her head and repeating my name urgently. I then noticed a strange burning vanilla smell, and it dawned on me, 'Oh my God, the eggs!' I leapt up, sprinted to the kitchen and quickly turned off the element. There was no water left in the pot and the whole house was smelling of burnt eggs. I'm the only person I know who has burnt boiled eggs. I sat there panicking about how I could have burnt the house down. I thought about living on my own and needing to be more alert. Then it occurred to me: Nan had woken me up. It feels weird talking about it, but she alerted me.

Caleb then explained to me that his grandmother had read our first book, *Tātaihono*. He recalled that one day he noticed that the book had disappeared off his bookshelf. He then discovered his grandmother reading it.

> I said to her, 'Who told you that you could read that?' Her response was, 'I can tell which one was your chapter!' I remarked, 'Well, that will teach you not to touch my things!' But it was clear to me that she loved it. Even though she wasn't very good at concentrating on reading and would only read a few pages at a time, she read the book cover to cover. She also related strongly to another chapter about a Cook Island family, something about a baby.

I told Caleb that the chapter was called, 'I Will Not Leave My Baby Behind'. Caleb continued,

> That story mattered to her because of her own experiences of being a Cook Island teenager in New Zealand and having a pregnancy and having her baby taken off her. I understood why that one was so meaningful for her. Even though she hardly ever talked about it, I know she was a spiritual person. After her own mother died, she told me she felt like her Mum never left her. She would go for walks or drives on her own, but she told me she never felt alone. She always felt like her mother was right next to her.

Since the incident with the burnt eggs, I am sometimes aware of my Nan's presence in the house. She is always standing just next to the table opposite where I usually sit. I find it hard to explain how I know that she is there, but it feels just like her. During her life, she had a big personality; she was loud and she loved colour. I feel like she comes because I am on my own and she is still here making sure that I am okay. When I feel her I can sense her breathing, and I realise that she is right here.

Wiremu

Although Caleb's Nan has physically died, it is clear to me from his kōrero that she has returned in spirit to help her moko (grandchild). People commonly report that experience of the breath, of hearing or feeling someone breathing, or of the sensation of breath on their skin. Such an experience on its own may not tell us if this is a good or bad spiritual presence. However, Caleb knows it's his Nan because she gives him that warm feeling. There is that feeling of aroha (love) in there. Perhaps that's one of the reasons people come back from beyond the veil to visit their loved ones. Perhaps she was lonely for him, too. So she has come back as his kaitiaki. And from Caleb's side, her death, his loneliness and his love for her may have contributed to this kūaha, this portal opening up just enough for him to be aware of her presence.

In Chapters 9 and 10 we have looked at two different approaches to assisting people who are experiencing voices and visions that they can't explain. Māori healing and psychiatric methods offer people very different forms of help and healing. When offered alongside each other, individuals and their whānau can benefit from both paradigms.

In this book, we have looked at multiple meanings of voices and visions. We have explored Māori and Western psychiatric views. Caleb's experiences are a reminder to us there are some things that science cannot explain. Here, Caleb has experiences of both seeing his Nan and hearing her voice. Perhaps a psychiatrist might say it could be his imagination, or a product of his mind caused by grief. Perhaps they might speculate that he was hallucinating because he was just waking up, when such experiences may be considered normal.

However, when I reflect on the nuances of Caleb's experiences, they demonstrate to me that wairua extends beyond the human body and beyond the death of the body. There is a saying, 'Ahakoa ka hinga te tinana, ka rere tonu te wairua'. Although the body falls, the spirit still soars.

Epilogue

Wiremu NiaNia and Allister Bush

This epilogue is an edited transcript of a wide-ranging conversation between Wiremu and Allister discussing their partnership and the way they work together.

Hīkoi Ngātahi

Allister: To finish off the book, our series editor, Art, suggested we add some dialogue between us about how we work together. You have often used the expression *Tātaihono* when referring to that. You talked of this as a kind of spiritual bond. To me this is quite a different description from the word 'bicultural', which is often used here in Aotearoa to describe services that bring together both Māori and Pākehā world views. How do you think about our partnership? What are your thoughts about other ways to describe how we have been doing this?

Wiremu: The problem I have with the word 'bicultural' is it comes from 'biculturalism', which is an imported word. I think it was invented by English- and French-speaking cultures in Canada. In Aotearoa it has been used by those in power when they were wanting to imply there was an equal relationship between Pākehā and Māori happening. But often there was nothing equal about it if you look at all the disparity.

I prefer to talk about hīkoi ngātahi. Hīkoi means a walk or journey and ngātahi suggests that we are plural but coming together. Hīkoi ngātahi suggests walking alongside each other as equals. For us it can mean collaboratively or cooperatively seeking the things that will benefit the people we work with.

Allister: So I guess the journey could have ups and downs.

Wiremu: Even though the journey might get bumpy, there's that thing of learning how to get through that together. There is also an emotional component to it. It's not a journey that's lightly taken just to

DOI: 10.4324/9781003187042-11

try it out. It's something that you may become emotionally attached to; that you might pour your heart into.

Allister: Okay, so you're talking about commitment.

Wiremu: Commitment, dedication. That makes it sound like you're going into a monastery!

Allister: Can there also be a playful element?

Wiremu: Yes. If you look at the way we have been on this hīkoi, we have had light times, we've enjoyed ourselves. We have also had many times when we seriously got down to working, trying to analyse what we were doing and figure out how we might improve our approaches to working with people. Other times we may throw in humour to help ward off things like getting grumpy because something is not going right. We have always found our way forward in difficult moments. So that's what hīkoi ngātahi means to me: being able to work things out together.

Allister: And get past the gnarly bits.

I have a question. It helps us to have a unified approach, but you and I also have our own separate perspectives. Do you think hīkoi ngātahi allows for that?

Wiremu: Well, there is an expression, 'whakaaro kotahi', which refers to thinking as one. Hīkoi ngātahi for me is different. It suggests we can have our diverse perspectives, but we are coming together.

Allister: We don't have to think as one.

Wiremu: Hell no!

Allister: I can hold on to my awareness that actually I'm coming from a very different perspective, and it helps me to be curious about what your views are, but not assume that I know. So many times I've assumed and I've been wrong.

Wiremu: Ngātahi means that we can lean on one another for understanding and to look at our different perspectives.

Racism and Trust

Wiremu: One question I have is did we have any hesitation working together? If we did, why the hesitation?

Allister: I assume you had some hesitation about working closely with a Pākehā like me. Can you comment on that?

Wiremu: Well, I went to a small rural school in Tiniroto. There were only three of us Māori kids at that school and about 20 Pākehā kids. We were in the middle of a farming community. Some of the older Pākehā kids called me black arse and [N-word]. I would get in fights most days with the kids who called me those names. When I was nine, we got a new principal who was also the only teacher.

He was English and he took an obvious dislike to me. He gave me a lot of hidings in the toilet over the three years he was at the school. He often hurt me, but he never left a mark on me, so it was hard to prove it. But what he did was hurt me psychologically as well. Those experiences had a lasting impression on me.

Allister: What effect do you think that had later?

Wiremu: Well, in my younger years, as an activist, there were times when I was full of anger. I talked about throwing Pākehā back into the sea!

Allister: Were there other experiences that affected you like that?

Wiremu: Lots of things. I remember going to the local store in Tiniroto. I would go up to the counter, and if a Pākehā walked into the shop, the shopkeeper used to ask me to stand to the side and wait till they were served. Often they would talk for ages and I had to leave because I had to get back to school. But she would always serve Pākehā first. There are plenty of other examples of racism. I didn't know what to call it in those days. For example, if a Māori turned up in a really nice car, the first thing some people would say was, 'Where did they pinch that from?'

I learnt to forgive that teacher many years later. I wish he was still alive so that I could tell him I forgive him to his face. Even though I never read the Bible, I like that saying, 'Do unto others as you would have them do unto you'.

Allister: What was your Nan's view on that?

Wiremu: My kuia was very spiritual. She would pray in the morning and pray at night. If we were going to town, she would pray that we would have a good trip, and everything would be safe. She always said 'Utua te kino ki te pai'. Bless those who would hurt you. I was to be the least of the least. Never raise myself above others.

Allister: What do you think she was getting at with that expression, 'Utua te kino ki te pai'?

Wiremu: That means always be slow to anger; that's what she meant. And it put us in good stead actually because it took me a very long time to get angry but when I did get angry, it took a quite a bit of stopping for me to settle down again.

Allister: I can understand that given what you experienced.

Wiremu: I notice that you haven't answered my question yet about what your hesitations were.

Allister: Well, I didn't have any hesitation working with you. I really wanted to do that once I realised a little of what you were doing. However, when you suggested we write about this work, one of my hesitations was that I didn't think that people would find my Pākehā viewpoint interesting. I also had doubts about what my psychiatrist colleagues would make of my involvement in this project. And I didn't expect readers would be interested in a mainstream psychiatry perspective from me.

Wiremu: That's the beauty of this! It's because we're walking alongside each other. One comes from the bush, the other is learned.

Allister: One is called Dr Bush.

Wiremu: [laughs] One is from the bush and the other is a Bush. And we come together and try to bring the best we can, out of each other and for the benefit of others.

Allister: I was really confident that your viewpoint would be interesting for people and very relevant for psychiatrists.

Wiremu: I think it's good for all of us to be able to look outside the box. We can get locked into our own viewpoints, eh?

Allister: Yeah. I was keen for people to see your explanations and perspectives clearly, and I presumed that the best way to do that would be to make mine invisible. Like getting out of the way.

Wiremu: I don't know about that. Because I think that was just as important.

Allister: Yeah, well you never let me get away with that. I recall you saying. 'If you're not going to tell your story, I won't tell my story either.'

In January 2010, I can remember you coming to the little office I was sitting in. You stood at the door and asked me, 'How about we write a book?' Over the previous weeks we had been having conversations about Caleb's situation. And because I had no clue about what writing a book would entail, I said – 'Oh yeah, okay'. I recall that after asking that, you added, 'But I need to let you know that I don't trust Pākehās'.

Wiremu: I think that was a cheeky comment.

Allister: But it was also about trust.

Wiremu: I think it was about being honest, that's what it was.

Allister: Why has that been important?

Wiremu: Well, we need to be transparent. So that we could have a better relationship.

Allister: I guess it could have been difficult between the two of us because I was a psychiatrist, and you were – I didn't know what you were.

Wiremu: [laughs] I didn't know what I was either!

Allister: What do you mean about that? What do you mean you didn't know what you were?

Wiremu: I didn't even know what I did well.

Allister: So you weren't seeing yourself as a tohunga?

Wiremu: No, I never ever saw myself as a tohunga.

Allister: But you were employed as a cultural therapist.

Wiremu: Yep.

Allister: So what did you see yourself as then?

Wiremu: Then I was just trying to define the role. I walked into something that was totally new for me.

Allister: What was it that was new?

Wiremu: Working in that clinical space was new. The role of cultural therapist was quite undefined. I was seeing things: that hadn't changed for me. But I didn't know if other kaimahi (clinicians) would believe that. I had to find ways to explain. Sometimes that shifted when I picked up something that was relevant to a person they were working with, which had not been talked about before.

Allister: You said something about – 'I don't trust you Pākehās', and you also said, 'I don't expect you to trust me either'. That was an important thing for us, being able to get past that and learn to trust each other.

Wiremu: Yeah, well for me it was simple. We clicked. That's wairua. It was okay. Being around you, I felt like I was in a safe space. As well as that, you were such an inquisitive blimmin' person. I liked the fact that you wanted to understand. I saw a willingness to learn, a genuine interest in our culture.

Working in Partnership

Wiremu: After we started having conversations, the next step in our collaboration was us doing sessions together with young people. We did sessions at Te Whare Mārie.

Allister: Yes, I remember I became very interested in sitting in with you. And you readily agreed.

Wiremu: I could see that you were curious about some of the stuff I was doing. I found it a lot easier to involve you rather than me having to explain. It was – what do you call it? Learning by being part of it. Rather than me having to describe it and break it down, you were able to see for yourself.

Allister: That led to further conversations. When I was in the middle of it and seeing some of what you are doing, I really did get curious because a lot of what you are doing, I didn't understand. And it wasn't even in any paradigm that I knew of. I had no way to think about it. No structure to help me make sense of it.

Wiremu: I knew that too. And when you would ask me, I wasn't struggling to give an answer, but I had that thing about the kūmara (sweet potato) not speaking about its own sweetness. [Proverb that Egan referred to in Chapter 5]. It was far better that you had a hands-on experience, right in the middle of it so you could figure it out.

Allister: But you know that kūmara thing, that really puzzled me. I had to talk to other people as well, like Egan. Because you were always so humble that made it very hard for me to understand some of the time what was going on. I found it easy to trust you though. You'd already been very helpful to me. You were kind. I had this feeling I could trust you, but it was a big mystery to me what you were doing.

Wiremu: Yeah, well same to me. I mean I knew I could see things but explaining that to clinicians, and knowing that people may or may not believe me was challenging.

Allister: What made that difference for you? How did you cross that threshold of learning to share some of this stuff?

Wiremu: I had a sense that you had your own spirituality. That let me know that you might be somebody who might listen to what I was saying about the unseen. Because it's not something you can easily share with people who may not believe you. I can tell by their expression on their face, they are thinking 'Oh what the heck!?' With you, that made it easier to open up a dialogue. So when you asked, 'Can we see a family together?' it was no problem to say 'Yeah'. And there was that thing of wairua saying it was okay. My trust in wairua.

Allister: So you felt like wairua was saying it was okay?

Wiremu: Yeah. 'It's okay'. If the spirit is in the right place, then you can go with it. If you have a check in the spirit, just one tiny check, then you should stop and pay attention to that. And that's not the logic part either; that's the spirit part. The mind is always suspicious. If the wairua is right, and it feels right, it is right.

Another part of learning to trust each other was not being afraid to question each other; to say, 'Hey, hang on a minute – what's this?' That mattered to me.

Allister: When you say, 'Hey – hang on a minute.' What do you mean?

Wiremu: I mean you and I can question each other about something the other one has said, if we are not sure about it. We could both trust that it would be received well. That there wouldn't be a defensive reaction. It would be more like, 'Oh, okay – tell me about it.' For me I can be confident to know that I can question and not create conflict. That's part of trust – that we know one another well enough to do that.

Allister: Yep – that's been really important.

Wiremu: Not that we've had to do that much recently, have we?

Allister: No, but I do think that trust has gotten much deeper over time.

Wiremu: At least we know that it's there if we need to use it. That's the thing, it's another tool in our kete. It makes for a good relationship because we always know that we can stay in our lanes, and if we need to, we can ask one another.

Allister: On the one hand, we are staying in our lanes, but on the other hand, we are interested in the other person's lane.

Wiremu: That's right, and there's nothing wrong with that.

Allister: For me developing our partnership has also been about acknowledging the history between us, between our cultures, and between our disciplines. We have to take account of that. This is not just you and me, working together as individuals. We're part of something that's gone before, and it wasn't always just and often it wasn't just.

Wiremu: But remember that you fellas were also colonised. So we can't only look at it that way.

Allister: Yep – like my Irish ancestors?

Wiremu: Yeah. Well, whoever it was. We were all colonised by one group or another so we can't really point fingers at anybody. I mean I'm the English as well: It's the black part of me! [laughs] I mean my grandfather is English. He came from Alveston I think. Wherever that is. So I can't point the finger. I can look at the injustices that happened. But it's the same blood, so I'm responsible as well.

Allister: Even though you've got such a generous perspective as that, it's still the case that there have been massive injustices, and you and I have talked a lot about finding a just approach; knowing that Māori healing was banned by law and psychiatry has been privileged. And all that stuff that you went through when you were young at primary school, I didn't have that. I went to a school where no one was telling me my culture was rubbish, I didn't get beaten for being Pākehā.

Wiremu: I can't imagine anyone calling you [N-word].

Allister: So there was a lot of privilege on my side. And I need to be aware of that.

Wiremu: Well, you also need to look at the fact that you might have missed out on something. Even with those abusive times, I gained a lot of experience. I gained a lot out of that emotionally. I learnt how I could be so angry that I wanted to kill somebody, and years later I reached a point when I felt so generous that I wanted to just go up and hug them. So I learnt some stuff out of it. And it stands me in good stead when I'm working now. That experience has taught me that I can be generous, and I tend to be generous most of the time.

Allister: I understand that and at the same time I wouldn't wish those experiences on anyone.

Wiremu: Well, I'm glad I had them, because it made me who I am.

Allister: But we also know that kind of injustice causes lots of grief and pain.

Wiremu: But even those experiences are worthwhile because now when I say to someone, 'I think I understand something of what you're going through', the thing is, I do have a clue. That could enable me to guide them through it. It gives me my own narrative I can relate to.

Allister: You've got something from that that you can use therapeutically.

Wiremu: Yeah, so I think I've gained an advantage.

Allister: But I'm still sure I don't wish these experiences on the younger generation or anyone. Those kinds of experiences have contributed to huge disadvantage for generations of people.

Wiremu: Yeah, that's fair enough. My mum couldn't speak English when she started school, and she got thrashed because she was speaking Māori. I know many others from that generation who did. And that happened to me and my generation as well. For many years I had a very different approach to this. I was totally into radical solutions. I was an activist. We fought for years and years to be heard, protesting against injustices like stolen Māori land and loss of our language. That was one way to make change, but it's not the only way. There is an expression, āhuru māwake, which refers to a gentle breeze. When it's blowing, people don't resist it. If it starts to become a squall, people may put barriers up. That's why more recently I have been interested in dialogue.

Allister: Dialogue might not always be comfortable, though. When we were in a wānanga (seminar) in Tūrangi before the pandemic, out of the blue you came up with this thing about me being like a Jack Russell terrier biting your ankles.

That was a joke but also it was talking about something in our relationship.

Wiremu: It talks about your tenacity. And your ferocity. When you sink your teeth into something you're not gonna let it go.

Allister: Even though I try to come across as a nice Pākehā?

Wiremu: Yeah, that's that pesky part of you that I notice. I actually think that's a term of endearment. There's a not giving up aspect. There is persistence. There is also something about loyalty there. That's a quality that I admire no matter what the situation. There is also something about our connection which meant I could bring that kind of humour into our kōrero. Sometimes that's how we've endeared ourselves to people. Making them laugh. Lightening it up for them for a moment. Not so much pressure for them to perform. But just relax and be who they are.

Allister: Well, I've noticed that happening in myself. Presenting with you, working with you, being around you.

Wiremu: It's something about humour that just takes a lot of weight off.

Writing this Book Together

Allister: Coming back to the topic of how we wrote this book, what would you say about that, because often we've gone over and over bits, haven't we?

Wiremu: Yep.

Allister: And so there is quite a lot of kōrero, and I've been often audiotaping conversations. How would you describe how we have done that?

Wiremu: I just thought it was natural. It's a natural way of learning. It's learning by saturation. And that's being right in the middle.

Allister: Learning by saturation?

Wiremu: Well, you know, when you're learning, getting things drummed into you, it's gotta sink in sooner or later, eh?

Allister: I think many times I have been very slow – it's taken ages for what you have said to sink in. But this general process, it is that related to the idea of wānanga?

Wiremu: Yes. That is wānanga. The thing about wānanga is it's not a lecture. We are all participants. When I'm participating, I can say what I think. I can offer my viewpoint. And other people can consider that, but they will also have their own perspectives. It gives you a broader view on one subject.

Allister: So I'm just thinking of all these conversations we've had which have ended up in this text. And then we've gone over the text together and you might have added a bit of extra kōrero, and I might have added a bit extra. I'm wondering how we explain this to people who don't know how we did it.

Wiremu: Well, the thing is, you and I are in wānanga all the time. And wānanga means sharing. It's not about one viewpoint. As opposed to following a book or a manual. We participate in the stuff we do. We both give to it; we both take away from it.

Allister: So we're taking away from it, and then having a chance to reflect.

Wiremu: Yes, that's right.

Allister: And then coming back together.

Wiremu: We can come back together and agree to change our approach.

Allister: Or have another exchange.

Wiremu: That's what we say in wānanga. What are you leaving behind? And what are you taking away? So I might leave behind my ignorance – that I didn't understand that particular topic, but I may take the best stuff that I could take away from here, and I'll add it to what I already have in order to enhance what I do.

Allister: Now you've got me thinking.

Wiremu: Well, I just hope that makes sense.

Allister: Is there anything in the root of wānanga that helps explain it?

Wiremu: The root of wānanga. 'Te wā' is the time, however long we have, it's the space, the season we do it in. 'Te wā' – is here and now. During that time, we are participating in kōrero. It's also the 'wa' in wairua. It's that stuff that transcends time and space. This allows us to reach back into the past to bring some stuff forward. So if you are in that space of wānanga – you are also in that space where wairua is. You have to give respect. When another person is speaking, we wait until they are finished. Whatever they say is tapu, sacred. It goes beyond just here – it's connected with the next dimension if you like.

Allister: Things that come out of wānanga may be inspired by wairua?

Wiremu: Yes

Allister: So if you can create space in wānanga for wairua, something special may come out.

Wiremu: Well, the thing with wānanga is that it starts with karakia, its starts with whanaungatanga – getting to know one another, finding the links to each other, bringing our ancestors together; it's that spiritual and physical bonding of sharing who you are and where you are from. Then the fact that you are participating. So the space of wānanga is everything that wairua is.

Allister: That's beautiful – and it brings us full circle to your kōrero in Chapter 1.

So maybe we can include this in our dialogue.

Wiremu: I will leave that to you, eh?

Allister: Okay.

Wiremu: I'm not clever enough.

Allister: Yeah, I would debate that, but I know I'm wasting my breath.

Finding the Good in People

Wiremu: Having come from my radical stance in the past, when I had so much anger toward Pākehā, in more recent decades I realised that even those who have hurt me are my fellow spiritual beings. For me that was like seeing the light. I decided I wanted to be the change myself, in order that any racist I might meet might have a possibility to learn something they didn't expect.

Allister: When you talk about light what are you meaning?

Wiremu: I think I was wanting to find the good in people. That everybody wasn't rotten. Everybody wasn't like the teacher who beat me at school.

Allister: One of the things I notice is that you frequently use biblical expressions – for example, early on in our kōrero here you referred to 'do unto others as you would have them do unto you'.

Wiremu: Yeah.

Allister: And just now you are talking about 'seeing the light'. Which you then describe as finding the good in people. Are you meaning that you view these things from a Christian point of view?

Wiremu: Could be, but not necessarily. I guess you can liken 'seeing the light' to getting up and seeing te atakura, which can be translated as the beautiful red glow of the breaking dawn, but at another level refers to your divine inner light. Another example is the expression 'Namaste' in Sanskrit, acknowledging that the light in me is also in you. It's no different to that. This spiritual concept is in many cultures.

Allister: Yes – and so on the one hand you're using biblical quotes and Christian metaphors and on the other hand you sometimes talk about Christianity as having a lot to answer for.

Wiremu: Yes it has! It *has* got a lot to answer for. It has attempted to take away people's beliefs, their culture and their identity, especially Māori and other Indigenous cultures. They've accused us of being idolaters, of talking to trees and talking to houses. When we get up and greet the whare (house), we say, 'Te whare e tū nei, tēnā koe'. And all we're saying is, this house that gives us warmth, that gives us shelter, we give thanks. We are giving thanks to the people who built it, who are no longer here. We're talking about whakapapa (genealogy), that gave the people who built this whare their lives, that we might be sheltered. And it's been misconstrued by the church and taken out of context, and they said that we're idolising all these different gods. See that's where I think Christianity was a form of trying to bring people into line.

Allister: So it contributed to colonisation.

Wiremu: It did. You can see this clearly in the Doctrine of Discovery, which I talked about in Chapter 4. This European legislation meant that Christian powers could take over any country that wasn't Christian and kill the people there. They could colonise any country they liked. People got killed in the name of God because they didn't believe in the same God. That's bloody terrible. So who are they to judge me and say, 'Oh, you sinner!' Hundreds of thousands of people died in the inquisitions. People were burned at the stake because they said hello to a cat. That's religiosity, it's legalistic and it's bloody rubbish.

Allister: At the same time I know that you are open to some parts of Christianity.

Wiremu: I'm open to it. I think it has some beautiful kōrero in it. Like – I've never read the Bible, but I know little things like 'do unto others ...' The beauty of that is, I don't have to think about how to express it, I can just say it and others will understand what I'm trying to say. But it doesn't mean to say I'm gonna go to church every blimmin' Sunday.

I love the people. At the same time, the church has been responsible for a lot of Māori being in conflict about their culture and whether it is even okay. I have a big problem with churches restricting people and directing them to reject their own cultures and identities. Those ideas are responsible for a lot of suffering and alienation for Indigenous people.

Presenting Together for the First Time

Allister: I remember the first time we presented together. I think it was 2009. The meeting was in a big room full of psychiatrists and other doctors, and you arrived after me. You knocked on the door and you opened it and peered into the room. I gestured to you to come in. As you entered in front of this large group, you suddenly gave a look of … I think you were hamming it up … but a fleeting look of horror flashed across your face as you eyeballed the audience.

Wiremu: I think that was real!

Allister: And then you made a joke, and everyone laughed. But what I noticed was that you felt okay there actually, you didn't look over-awed by that situation.

Wiremu: I tell you, years ago when I was in a band with my brothers, on the day we were performing I would make all the excuses in the world about why I should not take the front role leading the music. Or I would try to get out of singing and encourage one of my brothers to lead. But the thing is when they refused to take the lead, and I had to, once I got up on that stage, I became an entertainer.

Allister: Yes, I can imagine.

Wiremu: I was a stand-up comic, I could pull something humorous from anywhere, I could even make a joke about pūhā[1] growing in the area. For instance, 'I've noticed how big the pūhā is in this area and I would have brought a chainsaw to cut some if I'd known'. I could endear myself to people and every time I would say something, they would laugh. Often our whole night would go well because of that. I was always reluctant to start. I would try to get out of it if I could.

Allister: What do you think your reluctance was about?

Wiremu: Just not wanting to be up the front.

Allister: Do you remember that day when we were talking to the psychiatrists?

Wiremu: Now, whereabouts were we?

Allister: We were in the upstairs of the psychiatric unit at Wellington Hospital, and we were talking about Caleb's situation [from Chapter 1], and that morning I'd invited Caleb to come as well, and he texted me to say he had a job interview so he couldn't come.

Wiremu: Oh yeah, he was shy too.

Allister: Well, I didn't blame him for not coming. What was interesting was, I was really wondering if we or I would be criticised that day. There were a few key people in the audience who I thought would support us. What I noticed was that most of the psychiatrists in the audience seemed really curious, they were really interested in your point of view.

Wiremu: That's right.

Allister: And the way we presented it was 'Well, here's the story from the psychiatry point of view, but Wiremu, what do you think about this?'

Wiremu: Yeah, that's right.

Allister: And people really listened; they were really interested.

Wiremu: Well, they were curious.

Allister: Yeah, and you had some unique ways of explaining Māori concepts that were unfamiliar to them. And at question time, one of the things I wanted to do was to invite people to ask you the questions directly and they did. So that was part of the beginning of our dialogue.

Humour

Allister: I remember we did a talk one year and the Māori host introduced us as Wiremu NiaNia Tohunga and his sidekick, Allister Bush. I realised that day it was very hard for me to be in front of an audience and crack jokes. My natural tendency has been to be quite serious when talking in front of people. I really liked presenting with you because you often make people laugh. I made a comment that day about being the straight guy in this comedy duo and it certainly felt like that to me. I have often felt at ease being in front of an audience with you.

Wiremu: If I couldn't crack a joke, I wouldn't be able to stand up; otherwise, I'd be shaking too much.

Allister: Do you reckon making people laugh puts you at ease too?

Wiremu: Yep.

Allister: You know, I think we've done so many talks together, in some ways our relationship has developed in front of people.

Wiremu: I mean we couldn't help it. We worked together.

Allister: It's interesting how there's that element of performance. Because you and I are both musicians.

Wiremu: Well, I'm not, but you are.

Allister: Yeah well, you and Lesley [Wiremu's wife] are the ones who have been professional musicians.

Wiremu: I suppose I'm a lyricist or songwriter. I'm a romantic.

Allister: How many years were you singing in your band Te Mōkai for?

Wiremu: I believe in Robin Hood and all that sort of stuff.

Allister: I see you've artfully dodged my question. You mean robbing the rich to give to the poor?

Wiremu: Well, giving to the poor.

Allister: Looking after human beings, I think you mean.

Wiremu: Yep.

Allister: And not being too specific about what their background is.

Wiremu: I remember years ago, I was a diver. I would dive every second day and I would go into the community and drag a trailer load of kina (sea urchins) into the middle of the street and yell out 'Hey, bring your fellas' bowls!' and all these old people would come out of their whare and bring out their bowls. I would fill them up with kina and they would thank me so much, and I remember whenever I went down the street, they would offer me cups of tea.

Allister: Was that when you were doing youth work or before?

Wiremu: Well, I was still a rustler, so that must've been a long time ago. Perhaps when I was a teenager. I used to also take boot loads of meat in to feed people who couldn't afford to buy it.

Allister: Are you talking about in Gisborne?

Wiremu: Yeah. I knew the streets where the old people were.

Allister: Were you doing this by yourself or with your mates?

Wiremu: Whoever was with me at the time.

Allister: Those are good stories. I think I responded to that generosity as well. There is also generosity in the humour. I think that's been a big part of our relationship: you've always been so generous. And that positive feeling I can sense in the relationship. I know that's to do with wairua these days, but I wouldn't have had any words to put to that when we first met.

Music

Allister: Humour has been a big part. But there's something about music as well.

Wiremu: Yeah. Well, I'm not as musical as you guys. But there's something about music that attracts me, that draws me.

Allister: Yeah, I mean you might say that, but I see it differently – about how musical you are. But I remember seeing you and Lesley singing a beautiful waiata at Te Whare Mārie. Maybe it was in 2010.

It was a duet. And I remember thinking, 'Oh wow, that could go so well with a violin'.

Wiremu: [Laughs]

Allister: It must have been at someone's farewell, and I didn't know the meaning of the words or anything, but it was so beautiful. I never thought I'd get the opportunity to play it with you guys, because then you left Te Whare Mārie. Later on, we kept in touch, and then we had an opportunity of speaking at a conference together. We got talking about a waiata to go with our talk, and I asked, 'What was that song that you fellas did?' And when the two of you identified the waiata, I asked 'Could we do that one together?'

I play the violin, and my training was classical, which I never thought would fit in with you and Lesley …

Wiremu: … with Māori kupu, with Māori songs.

Allister: But you guys immediately thought it would fit. I was quite shy about it. It took me by surprise. It took me a while to get my head around it. However, as soon as we started talking about it, you guys said, 'Let's do it'. Lesley was saying 'Come on, Allister, get your violin out', then 'Right! Here are the notes you've got to play.' Then she just sang it. She was making up the harmony on the spot. I wasn't used to playing without sheet music. So I was busy scribbling out the notes and saying, 'Lesley, stop … I need to write it down'. It took me ages to learn it off by heart, over the many times we performed that waiata together.

It was only later that you explained the kupu to me. How would you explain the meaning of that song?

Wiremu: That waiata is 'Whakapipiri mai', which we call 'Kaua e whai mai'. It was by Dave Henere and Huia Reweti. The meaning of the kupu is, 'Do not follow for I may not lead, do not lead for I may not follow. Instead, please walk beside me and be my friend.' When I'm singing, the emotion in the waiata is most important to me. If it has no feeling for me then I don't bother to do it. The relationship and the emotions are part and parcel of that waiata. If you express something genuinely when you're singing the waiata and if you express it emotionally, it means a hell of a lot more to the people listening. Even if you're flat as and you forget the words, because you've endeared yourself to those people it doesn't matter.

Allister: When we performed it, you've talked about it as a metaphor for collaboration.

Wiremu: Yes, you see, that's the beauty of it. If we look at it poetically, if we look at the imagery in the waiata, it's all there, the words, the emotion, everything is in that song.

Allister: How do you see that as relevant to our partnership?
Wiremu: Oh, it means let neither one of us walk up in front, do not be the follower, but let's do this together – that's what that song means.
Allister: That makes sense to me. It feels like you and I have done that, to the best of our ability.

Note

1 Sow thistle, considered a green leafy delicacy, often used in a boil up stew.

Glossary

ā wairua	pertaining to the spiritual realm
Ahakoa ka hinga te tinana, ka rere tonu te wairua	although the body falls, the spirit still soars
āhua	appearance
āhuru māwake	gentle breeze
aiga (Samoan)	family
Aotearoa	Māori name for New Zealand
apa	spirit of an ancestor, angel(s), heavenly being(s)
aro	to give attention to
aroha	love, respect, compassion
atua	ancestor(s), supernatural being(s), deity/deities
awa	river(s)
awhi	to embrace, cherish, support
fa'asamoa (Samoan)	Samoan worldview
fono (Samoan)	meeting
hā	breath
haka	Māori cultural ritual with energetic rhythmical actions and words, embodying a mana-enhancing expression of identity and unity
Hauhau	Māori movement founded in 1862 to fight against unjust confiscation of land
he aha te pūtake?	what is the root cause?
hīnātore	glimmer of light
hinengaro	mind, psychological
Hine-pūkohu-rangi	goddess of mist, ancestress of Ngāi Tūhoe nation
Hinewai	goddess of light misty rain, sister of Hine-pūkohu-rangi
hōhā	irritated, annoyed, annoying
hōiho	horse
hua	fruit, product

huakina	to open
hui	gathering, meeting, to meet
Ihoa/Ihowā	Jehovah, God
Io	supreme being, God
iwi	tribe, people, nation
kahupō	to be clothed or cloaked in darkness
kai	food, meal
kaimahi	clinician(s) or worker(s)
kaimoana	sea food, fisheries
kāinga	home, village(s)
kaitiaki	guardian(s), spiritual guardian(s)
kākahu	clothing
Ka kuhu tonu ia	refers to the ability to do things your way, in your time.
kanohi ki te kanohi	face to face
kapa haka	Māori cultural performance
karakia	ritual chant(s), prayer(s), customary blessing
karanga	ceremonial call of welcome
kaua e whai mai	do not follow me
kaupapa	purpose
kaupapa Māori	Māori approach, Māori centred
kaumātua	elder(s), a person of status in the family
kēhua	ghost, apparition
Kei te rongo au te kakara o te kai	I can hear the fragrance of the food
kēkē	the hollow part of the armpit
kete	basket(s)
kia tau	let it settle
kina	sea urchins
koha	gift, offering, donation
kōhanga reo	Māori language preschool
kōrero	talk, conversation, explanation
koro	grandfather, term of respect to address an elderly man
koroua	male elder(s)
korowai	cloak, cloak of protection
kū	keening sound, inarticulate sound
kuhu	to go inside to work something out
kuia	female elder, grandmother
kūmara	sweet potato
kumu	anus, buttocks
kupu	word(s)
kūwaha	mouth
mahi	work
māhunga	head

mamae	hurt, pain
mana	authority, spiritual authority
manaaki	support, hospitality, to protect, to take care of
manuhiri	visitor(s)
mānuka	native scrub tree with aromatic foliage, tea tree
Māori	Indigenous person/people of Aotearoa (New Zealand)
marae	ceremonial meeting house. Also, the open area in front of the meeting house where formal greetings and discussions take place
marama	moon
maro	garment resembling short kilt
mata	face
Mātaatua	great migration waka (canoe) captained by Toroa, which is the ancestral waka of Ngāi Tūhoe and other iwi (tribes) in Northland and Bay of Plenty
matakite	seer, foresight
mataora	full facial male Māori tattoo
mātauranga	knowledge
mātauranga Māori	Māori knowledge
matekite	spiritual awareness, seer, insight into the spiritual realm
matekitetanga	everything pertaining to a person's matekite gift
matekite wānanga	spiritual awareness workshops
mate Māori	Māori sickness or illness
Matike Mai	to rise up; the name of an independent working group promoting constitutional transformation in Aotearoa
matū	the gist, the substance of a matter
matua	parent, uncle, respectful way to address male elder
maunga	mountain, ancestral mountain
Maungapōhatu	ancestral mountain of Ngāi Tūhoe
mauri	life force
me kuhu koe i a koe tonu	one should go into oneself to look for the answers
me whakaiti koe i a koe	you must always be the least
mihimihi	greeting, speech(es) of greeting
mimi	to urinate, pee
moana	ocean
moemoeā	dreams
moko	grandchild; also, art of Māori tattooing

mokopuna	grandchild
Moriori	the Indigenous people of Rēkohu, the Chatham Islands
Ngā Kūaha	doorways, entranceways
ngā mōrehu	the survivors
Ngāi Tūhoe	the Tūhoe peoples
ngāngara	insect(s), reptile(s) or creepy-crawlies
ngā poropiti	prophets
ngā taonga tuku iho	precious knowledge handed down from ancestors
ngā tōpito o te ao	the farthest places of the earth
ngatoroirangi	the fires of heaven
ngāwari	patient, affable, easygoing, flexible
noho puku	to remain silent, an attitude of holding one's experience inside and keeping it to oneself
nono	anus, backside, butt
Ole Taeao Afua (Samoan)	The New Morning, name given to a Samoan study on mental health
Palagi (Samoan)	New Zealand European, European
Pākehā	New Zealand European
pakeke	adult
Pakerewha	The prophet Toiroa used this expression to refer to the coming of strangers who brought disease
Papa	respectful way to address older male
Papatūānuku	earth mother
patupaiarehe	fairy folk
pēpē	baby
piupiu	ceremonial garment made of flax, worn between waist and knees
pīwakawaka	fantail
ponga	tree fern
poroaki	ceremonial farewell
pounamu	New Zealand greenstone or jade, greenstone pendant or precious object
pōuri	sad, disheartened
pōwhiri	ceremonial welcome
pūhā	sowthistle, green leafy delicacy often used in boil up stews
pūkoro	pocket, also used by the prophet Toiroa to refer to a garment resembling trousers
puku	stomach
pūrākau	Māori narrative(s)
pūtake	root cause, origin
rākau	ceremonial staff, may symbolise authority to speak

rangatahi	youth, younger generation
rangatira	leader(s), female or male chief(s)
Ranginui	sky father
Rata	a hero of Māori cultural narratives
reka	sweetness
Rēkohu	Wharekauri, the Chatham Islands
rerekētanga	something that's different
rēwena	sourdough potato bread
rimu	large native forest trees with gracefully weeping foliage
rohe	area
rōpū	group
rongoā	medicine
rua	receptacle, container, knowledge, also means two
Rūaumoko	atua of earthquakes and volcanoes, youngest offspring of Papatūānuku and Ranginui
taha wairua	spiritual side or part
taiaha	long wooden Māori weapon, Māori martial art
taihoa	wait
tairongo	sense(s), intuition
takahi	to trample on, to disregard
tamaiti	child
tamariki	children
tāne	man, male, husband
Tāne-mahuta	atua of forests and birds, one of the offspring of Papatūānuku and Ranginui
tangata	person
tāngata	people
tāngata whaiora	seekers of wellbeing
tangihanga	bereavement ritual
taonga	something precious which may be tangible or intangible
tapu	to be sacred, restricted or forbidden
tarutaru	cannabis
tātaihono	spiritual binding together that confers unity and strength to a partnership
taupopoki	the prophet Toiroa used this expression to refer to a head covering or hat
tautoko	support
te ao Māori	the Māori world
te ao mārama	the world of light, enlightenment
te ao Pākehā	the Pākehā world
te ao tawhito	times of old
te ao wairua	the spiritual realm
te atakura	red glow of breaking dawn, also divine inner light
te Hāhi Ringatū	the Ringatū faith

teina	younger sibling of same gender
teka	false, lie(s)
Te Kaihanga	the Creator, God
Te Kore	the void, realm of potential being
Tekau mā rua	the 12th day of the month in Ringatū faith
Te Korokoro-o-te-parata	a dangerous whirlpool
Te Māngai	the mouthpiece
Te Moana-nui-a-Kiwa	The Pacific Ocean
tēnei te pō, nau mai te ao	at our darkest moments, we may find the light we need
Te Pō	impenetrable darkness
te reo	Māori language
Te Urewera	the rohe (ancestral area) of Ngāi Tūhoe
Te Waonui a Tāne	the great forest of Tāne
Te Whare Mārie	literally, the house of peace: Māori mental health service based in Porirua
Te Tiriti o Waitangi	The Treaty of Waitangi
tika	correct
tikanga	correct procedure or convention, usually referring to Māori customs
tinana	physical, body
tino rangatiratanga	unqualified authority, sovereignty
tipuna, tīpuna	ancestor(s), same as tupuna, tūpuna
tiro	to observe or examine
tirohanga	view(s)
titipa	striped earthworm
titiro	to look, observe, examine
tohunga	Māori healer or expert
tohungatanga	practices and knowledge pertaining to Māori expertise
tohunga wairua	Māori spiritual healer
tokotoko	staff
Toroa	captain of the Mātaatua waka (ancestral canoe)
tōtara	large native forest trees
tuakana	older sibling of same gender
tūpāpaku	body of the deceased
tūrehu	spiritual creatures that are part human and part animal
Tūranganui-a-Kiwa	literally 'the great standing place of Kiwa', Māori name for 'Poverty Bay', area around Gisborne
tūrangawaewae	family land, place of belonging through kinship, place to stand

Uenuku	a mortal who fell in love with the goddess Hine-pūkohu-rangi, rainbow
Uepoto	one of the offspring of Papatūānuku and Ranginui, the first to see light
urupā	cemetery, burial ground
utu	reciprocity, cost, exchange
utua te kino ki te pai	bless those who would hurt you
waha	mouth, entrance
wāhine	women
waiata	song(s)
waikahu	amniotic fluid
waiora	healing water, health
Wairua	Divine Source
wairua	spiritual, spirituality, spiritual realm, spirit
wairuatanga	the spiritual dimension
waka	canoe, ancestral canoe, vessel
wānanga	seminar, forum, group learning setting
whakaiti	to make small, self-effacing
whakaaro	ideas
whakamā	shame, embarrassment
whakamana	acknowledge the mana or authority of a person, family or group
whakamomori	to internalise grief, desperation, to contemplate a desperate act or suicide
whakapapa	genealogy
whakapipiri mai	draw closer to me
whakatau	formal welcome
whakatauākī	proverb
whakawetewete	ritual to release anger, unresolved hurt, or resolve conflict, or transgressions between people
whāngai	extended family adoption
whānau	family
whanaungatanga	kinship, relationship
whare	house
Wharekauri	the Chatham Islands, Rēkohu
wharepaku	toilet
whare tangata	house of people, womb
whare wānanga	school of Māori healing, university, place of higher learning
whenua	land, also afterbirth or placenta

References

American Psychiatric Association. (1994). *Diagnostic and statistical manual of mental disorders* (4th edition). American Psychiatric Publishing.

American Psychiatric Association, DSM-5 Task Force. (2013). *Diagnostic and statistical manual of mental disorders: DSM-5* (5th edition). American Psychiatric Publishing.

Belich, J. (1996). *Making peoples – A history of the New Zealanders*. Penguin.

Benton, R., Frame, A., & Meredith, P. (Eds.). (2013). *Te Mātāpunenga: A compendium of references to the concepts and institutions of Māori customary law*. Victoria University Press.

Berrios, G. E. (1990). A theory of hallucinations: Auguste Tamburini. *History of Psychiatry, 1*, 145–150.

Berrios, G. E. (1996). *The history of mental symptoms: Descriptive psychopathology since the nineteenth century*. Cambridge University Press.

Best, E. (1972). *Tuhoe: The children of the mist*. (Volume 1, 2nd edition). Reed.

Bidois, E. (2017). Tahi. *Mad in Aotearoa*. Retrieved from: https://madinaotearoa/2017/02/27/tahi-egan-bidois/

Bidois, E. (2019). Angels and Demons (Episode 1). In *Out of My Mind: True stories about mental health, told by people who've been there*. Retrieved from: https://interactives.stuff.co.nz/2019/08/out-of-my-mind-podcast/angels-and-demons on 11 October, 2021. Stuff Podcast.

Binney, J. (1990). Ancestral Voices: Māori prophet leaders. Chapter 7 in Sinclair, K., ed. *The Oxford illustrated history of New Zealand*. Oxford University Press.

Binney, J. (1995). *Redemption songs: A life of the nineteenth-century Maori leader Te Kooti Arikirangi Te Turuki*. University of Hawai'i Press.

Binney, J., Chaplin, G., & Wallace, C. (1979). *Mihaia: The Prophet Rua Kenana and his community at Maungapohatu*. Oxford University Press.

Bleuler, E. (1950). *Dementia praecox or the group of schizophrenias*. International Universities Press. (Original work published in German in 1911)

Braun, C. M., Dumont, M., Duval, J., et al. (2003). Brain modules of hallucination: An analysis of multiple patients with brain lesions. *Journal of Psychiatry & Neuroscience, 28*, 432–449.

Brewin, C. R., & Patel, T. (2010). Auditory pseudohallucinations in United Kingdom war veterans and civilians with posttraumatic stress disorder. *Journal of Clinical Psychiatry, 71*(4), 419–425.

Bush, A., & NiaNia, W. (2012). Voice hearing and pseudoseizures in a Māori Teenager: An example of Mate Māori and Māori traditional healing. *Australasian Psychiatry, 20*, 348–351.

Castor, H. (2014). *Joan of Arc: A history*. Faber & Faber.
Chow, W. S., & Priebe, S. (2013). Understanding psychiatric institutionalization: A conceptual review. *BMC Psychiatry, 13*, 169.
Coleman, R. (1999). *Recovery: An alien concept*. Handsell Press.
Cook, C. C. H. (2013). Recommendations for psychiatrists on spirituality and religion. Position Statement PS03/2013. Royal College of Psychiatrists.
Cook, C. C. H., Powell, A., & Sims, A. (Eds.). (2009). *Spirituality and psychiatry*. Royal College of Psychiatrists.
Department of Internal Affairs. (2007). *Te Āiotanga: Report of the Confidential Forum for Former in-Patients of Psychiatric Hospitals*.
Dillon, J., & May, R. (2002). Reclaiming experience. *Clinical Psychology, 17*, 25–27.
dos Santos, L. (2007). *Fatima in Lucia's own words: Sister Lucia's memoirs*. Secretariado Dos Pastorinhos.
Durie, M. (1998). *Whaiora: Māori health development* (2nd edition). Oxford University Press.
Durie, M. (2011). Indigenizing mental health services: New Zealand experience. *Transcultural Psychiatry 48*, 24–36.
Elkington, B., Jackson, M., Kiddle, R., et al. (2020). *Imagining decolonisation*. Bridget Williams Books.
Elsaesser, E., Roe, C. A., Cooper, C. E., & Lorimer, D. (2021). The phenomenology and impact of hallucinations concerning the deceased. *British Journal of Psychiatry Open, 16*, 7.
Flanagan, S. (1998). *Hildegard of Bingen – A visionary life* (2nd edition). Routledge.
Foxhall, K. (2014). Making modern migraine medieval: Men of science, Hildegard of Bingen and the life of a retrospective diagnosis. *Medical History, 58*(3), 354–374.
Grace, P. (1992). *Cousins*. Penguin.
Gutkovich, D. (2020). *Life with voices: A guide for harmony*. Life with Voices.
Holman, J. (2010). *Best of both worlds: The story of Elsdon Best and Tutakangahau*. Penguin.
Huirama, T. (2019). *Walking with Tūpuna: Gathering our light*.
Ihimaera, W. (2020). *Navigating the stars: Māori creation myths*. Penguin Random House.
James, W. (2002). *The varieties of religious experience: A study in human nature*. The Modern Library. (Original work published in 1902).
Kapur, S. (2003). Psychosis as a state of aberrant salience: A framework linking biology, phenomenology, and pharmacology in schizophrenia. *American Journal of Psychiatry, 160*, 13–23.
Kauffman, P., & McLennan, R. (2017). Did schizophrenia exist in ancient Greece and Rome?: Schizophrenia and epigenetics. *The International Journal of Health, Wellness and Society, 7*(4), 9–23.
King, M. (1989). *Moriori: A people rediscovered*. Viking.
Kingi, T. K., Durie, M., Elder, H., et al. (2017). *Maea Te Toi Ora: Māori health transformations*. Huia.
Kraepelin, E. (1919). *Dementia praecox and paraphrenia* (trans. R. M. Barclay, G. M. Robertson, ed.). Robert Krieger. (Original work published in German in 1896.)
Larøi, F., Luhrmann, T. M., Bell, V., et al. (2014). Culture and hallucinations: Overview and future directions. *Schizophrenia Bulletin, 40*(Supplement 4), S213–20.
Leff, J., Sartorius, N., Jablensky, A., et al. (1992). The international pilot study of schizophrenia: Five-year follow-up findings. *Psychological Medicine, 22*(1), 131–145.

Leudar, I., & Thomas, P. (2000). *Voices of reason, voices of insanity: Studies of verbal hallucinations*. Routledge.

Longden, E. (2010). Making sense of voices: A personal story of recovery. *Psychosis: Psychological, Social and Integrative Approaches, 2*(3), 255–259.

Longden, E., Read, J., & Dillon, J. (2018). Assessing the impact and effectiveness of hearing voices network self-help groups. *Community Mental Health Journal, 54*, 184–188.

Luhrmann, T. M. (2012). *When God talks back: Understanding the American Evangelical Relationship with God*. Knopf.

Luhrmann, T. M. (2017). Diversity within the psychotic continuum. *Schizophrenia Bulletin, 43*(1), 27–31.

Luhrmann, T. M., Ramachandran, P., Tharoor, H., & Osei, A. (2015). Differences in voice-hearing experiences of people with psychosis in the USA, India and Ghana: Interview-based study. *British Journal of Psychiatry, 206*, 41–44.

Mair, G. (1923). *Reminiscences and Maori stories*. Brett Publishing.

Maj, M. (2018). Why the clinical utility of diagnostic categories in psychiatry is intrinsically limited and how we can use new approaches to complement them. *World Psychiatry, 17*, 121–122.

Manford, M., & Andermann, F. (1998). Complex visual hallucinations: Clinical and neurobiological insights. *Brain, 121*, 1819–1840.

Matike Mai Aotearoa. (2016). He Whakaaro Here Whakaumu mō Aotearoa. *The report of Matike Mai Aotearoa- the independent working group on constitutional transformation*.

Matua Raki. (2009). *Takarangi competency framework: Ngā Pukenga Ahurea*.

McCarthy-Jones, S. (2012). *Hearing voices: The histories, causes and meanings of auditory verbal hallucinations*. Cambridge University Press.

McCarthy-Jones, S., & Longden, E. (2015). Auditory verbal hallucinations in schizophrenia and post-traumatic stress disorder: Common phenomenology, common cause, common interventions? *Frontiers in Psychology, 6*, 1–12.

McGorry, P. (2015). Early intervention in psychosis: Obvious, effective, overdue. *The Journal of Nervous and Mental Disease, 203*, 310–318.

McLeod, M., King, P., Stanley, J. et al. (2017). Ethnic disparities in the use of seclusion for adult psychiatric inpatients in New Zealand. *New Zealand Medical Journal, 130*, 30–39.

Mikaere, B. (1988). *Te Maiharoa and the promised land*. Reed.

Mila-Schaaf, K. (2010). Keynote address at Building Bridges Conference, Wellington. Retrieved from: https://hearingvoices.org.nz/index.php/en/personal-stories/44-giving-voice-to-the-voidby-karla-mila-schaaf

Ministry of Health. (2012). *Rising to the challenge: The mental health and addiction service development plan 2012–2017*.

Mitchell, P. (2011). Retrospective diagnosis and the use of historical texts for investigating disease in the past. *International Journal of Paleopathology, 1*, 81–88.

Mohatt, G., & Eagle Elk, J. (2000). *The price of a gift: A Lakota healer's story*. University of Nebraska Press.

Moon, P. (2003). *Tohunga: Hohepa Kereopa*. David Ling Publishing.

Moreira-Almeida, A., Sharma, A., van Rensburg, B. J., et al. (2016). WPA position statement on spirituality and religion in psychiatry. *World Psychiatry, 15*(1), 87–88.

Morse, G., & García, M. (2021). Dreams, visions and hallucinations with Indigenous populations: Ethical considerations. Chapter 2 in G. Morse, & V. Lomay (Eds.), *Understanding Indigenous perspectives: Visions, dreams, and hallucinations*. Cognella.

Moseley, P., Powell, A., Woods, A., et al. (2022). Voice-hearing across the continuum: A phenomenology of spiritual voices. *Schizophrenia Bulletin, 48*(5), 1066–1074.

Muramoto, O. (2014). Retrospective diagnosis of a famous historical figure: Ontological, epistemic and ethical considerations. *Philosophy, Ethics, and Humanities in Medicine, 9*, 10. Retrieved from: http://www.peh-med.com/content/9/1/10

Murray, T. D. (1902). *Jeanne D'Arc: Maid of Orleans – Deliverer of France*. McClure Phillips.

Newman, B. (1985). Hildegard of Bingen: Visions and validation. *Church History, 54*(2), 163–175.

Newman, K. (2009). *Ratana the Prophet*. Penguin.

Ngata, R. (2014). *Understanding matakite: A Kaupapa Māori study on the impact of Matakite/Intuitive experiences on wellbeing*. Doctoral Thesis. Massey University.

Ngata, T. (2019). *Kia Mau: Resisting colonial fictions*.

NiaNia, W., Bush, A., & Epston, D. (2017a). *Collaborative and indigenous mental health therapy: Tātaihono – Stories of Māori healing and psychiatry*. Routledge.

NiaNia, W., Bush, A., & Epston, D. (2019). He korowai o ngā tīpuna: Voice hearing and communication from ancestors. *Australasian Psychiatry, 27*, 345–347.

NiaNia, W., Mana, Rangi, Bush, A., & Epston, D. (2017b) Restoring mana and taking care of Wairua: A story of Māori Whānau healing. *Australian and New Zealand Journal of Family Therapy, 38*, 72–97.

NiaNia, W., Tere, Bush, A., & Epston, D. (2013). 'I will not leave my baby behind': A Cook Island Māori family's experience of New Zealand Māori traditional healing. *Australian and New Zealand Journal of Family Therapy, 34*, 3–17.

O'Hagan, M. (2015). *Madness made me: A memoir*. Potton & Burton.

Osis, K., & Haraldsson, E. (1977). *At the hour of death*. Avon.

Otago Daily Times (2010). Coroner issues finding on death of Janet Moses. August 12th, Dunedin. Accessed at: odt.co.nz/news/national/coroners-issues-finding-death-janet-moses on 22 January, 2023.

Owen, A. (1989). *The darkened room: Women, power, and spiritualism in late Victorian England*. Virago Press.

Oyebode, F. (2018). *Sims' symptoms in the mind: Textbook of descriptive psychopathology* (6th edition). Elsevier.

Penfield, W., & Perot, P. (1963). The brain's record of auditory and visual experience. *Brain, 86*(4), 595–696.

Plato. (1993). *The last days of Socrates*. (Trans. H. Tredennick and H. Tarrant, 1954). Penguin. (Original work in Greek, 395BC)

Poole, R., Cook, C. C. H., & Higgo, R. (2019). Psychiatrists, spirituality and religion. *British Journal of Psychiatry, 214*(4), 181–182.

Rangihuna, D., Kopua, M., & Tipene-Leach, D. (2018). Mahi a Atua: A pathway forward for Māori mental health? *New Zealand Medical Journal, 131*, 79–83.

Roxburgh, E. C., & Roe, C. A. (2014). Reframing voices and visions using a spiritual model. An interpretative phenomenological analysis of anomalous experiences in mediumship. *Mental Health Religion and Culture, 17*(6), 641–653.

Royal, T. A. C. (Ed.). (2003). *The woven universe: Selected writings of Rev. Māori Marsden*. The Estate of Rev. Māori Marsden.

S.L. (1953). *The boy who saw true*. C.W. Daniel.

Sackeim, H. A. (2017). Modern electroconvulsive therapy: vastly improved yet greatly underused. *JAMA Psychiatry*; 74(8), 779–780.

Sadock, B., & Sadock, V. (Eds.). (2005). *Kaplan and Sadock's comprehensive textbook of psychiatry* (8th edition). Lippincott, Williams & Wilkins.

Saint Teresa of Ávila. (1957). *The life of Saint Teresa of Ávila* (Trans. J. Cohen). Penguin. (Original work in Spanish, 1588)

Schildkrout, B. (2017). Joan of Arc – Hearing voices. *American Journal of Psychiatry, 174*(12), 1153–1154.

Schneider, K. (1959). *Clinical psychopathology*. (trans. M. W. Hamilton). Grune & Stratton. (original work in German)

Scholz, B., Gordon, S., & Happell, B. (2017). Consumers in mental health service leadership: A systematic review. *International Journal of Mental Health Nursing, 26*, 20–31.

Shapiro, F. (2001). *Eye movement desensitization and reprocessing: Basic principles, protocols, and procedures* (2nd edition). Guilford.

Sidgwick, H., Johnson, A., Myers, F. W. H., et al. (1894). Report on the census of hallucinations. *Proceedings of the Society for Psychical Research, 10*, 25–422.

Sims, A. (1995). *Symptoms in the mind: An introduction to descriptive psychopathology* (2nd edition). Saunders.

Sinha, R. (2021). Charles VI of France: The glass king. *British Journal of Psychiatry, 218*, 50.

Skodlar, B., & Jørgensen, J. P. (2013). Could Socrates be diagnosed within the schizophrenia spectrum? Could schizophrenia patients be considered in the light of Socratic insights? *Psychosis, 5*(1), 17–25.

Smith, L. T. (2012). *Decolonizing methodologies: Research and Indigenous peoples* (2nd edition). Otago University Press.

Soares-Weiser, K., Maayan, N., Bergman, H., et al. (2015). First rank symptoms for schizophrenia. *Cochrane Database of Systematic Reviews, 1*, CD010653.

Spittles, B. (2022). *Psychosis, psychiatry and psychospiritual considerations: Engaging and better understanding the madness and spiritual emergence nexus*. Aeon Books.

Stace, H. (2019). Statement of Hilary Stace to the Royal Commission of Inquiry into historical abuse in state care and in the care of faith-based institutions: Contextual public hearing.

Stahl, S. M. (2013). *Stahl's essential psychopharmacology: Neuroscientific basis and practical application* (4th edition). Cambridge University Press.

Stirling, E., & Salmond, A. (1980). *Eruera: The teachings of a Maori elder*. Oxford University Press.

Tamasese, K., Peteru, C., & Waldegrave, C. (1997). *Ole Taeao Afua: A qualitative investigation into Samoan perspectives on mental health and culturally appropriate services. Report for the Health Research Council of New Zealand*. The Family Centre.

Tamasese, K., Peteru, C., Waldegrave, C., & Bush, A. (2005). Ole Taeao Afua, the new morning: A qualitative investigation into Samoan perspectives on mental health and culturally appropriate services. *Australian and New Zealand Journal of Psychiatry 39*, 300–309.

Thatikonda, P. S. (2019). Spirituality in psychiatry practice. *Indian Journal of Psychological Medicine, 41*(2), 103–107.

Theuma, M., Read, J., Moskowitz, A., & Stewart, A. (2007). Evaluation of a New Zealand early intervention service for psychosis. *New Zealand Journal of Psychology, 36*, 136–145.

Tien, A. Y. (1991). Distributions of hallucinations in the population. *Social Psychiatry and Psychiatric Epidemiology, 26*, 287–292.

van den Berg, D. P. G., de Bont, P. A. J., Berber, M., et al. (2015). Prolonged exposure vs Eye movement desensitization and reprocessing vs Waiting list for post-traumatic stress disorder in patients with a psychotic disorder: A randomized clinical trial. *JAMA Psychiatry, 72*(3), 259–267.

van der Hart, O., Nijenhuis, E. R. S., & Solomon, R. (2010). Dissociation of the personality in complex trauma-related disorders and EMDR: Theoretical considerations. *Journal of EMDR Practice and Research, 4*(2), 76–92.

Viana, M., Tronvik, E. A., Do, T. P., et al. (2019). Clinical features of visual migraine aura: A systematic review. *Journal of Headache and Pain, 20*(1), 64, 1–7.

Waitangi Tribunal. (2009). *Te Urewera: Pre-publication – Part 1.* (WAI 894).

Waitoki, W., & Levy, M. (Eds.). (2016). *Te Manu Kai i Te Mātauranga: Indigenous psychology in Aotearoa/New Zealand.* New Zealand Psychological Society.

Waldegrave, C., Tamasese, K., Tuhaka, F., & Campbell, W. (2003). *Just therapy - A journey: A collection of papers from the just therapy team, New Zealand.* Dulwich Centre Publications.

Walker, R. (2004). *Ka Whawhai Tonu Matou: Struggle without end.* Penguin.

Waters, F., Blom, J. D., Dang-Vu, T. T., et al. (2016). What is the link between hallucinations, dreams and hypnagogic-hypnopompic experiences? *Schizophrenia Bulletin, 42*(5), 1098–1109.

Waters, F., Collerton, D., Ffytche, D. H., et al. (2014). Visual hallucinations in the psychosis spectrum and comparative information from neurodegenerative disorders and eye disease. *Schizophrenia Bulletin*, vol. 40 suppl. no. 4, S233–S245.

Wayman, D. (1957). The chancellor and Jeanne D'Arc: February – July AD 1429. *Franciscan Studies, 17*, 273–305.

Williams, H. (2022, August). Veteran Māori broadcaster, artist and teacher Haare Williams [Interview] Radio New Zealand. Retrieved from: https://www.rnz.co.nz/national/programmes/mapuna/audio/2018856059/veteran-maori-broadcaster-artist-and-teacher-haare-williams

Young, D. (1998). *Woven by water: Histories from the Whanganui river.* Huia.

Index

Pages followed by "n" refer to notes.